A Colour Atlas of
Clinical
Gynaecology

V. R. Tindall
MD MSc FRCS FRCOG
Professor of Obstetrics and Gynaecology
University of Manchester

Wolfe Medical Publications Ltd

A Colour Atlas of Clinical Gynaecology

Copyright © V. R. Tindall, 1981
Published by Wolfe Medical Publications Ltd, 1981
Printed by Smeets-Weert, Holland
ISBN 0 7234 0761 4 Cased edition
ISBN 0 7234 1551 X Paperback edition
Paperback edition, © 1988

A CIP catalogue record for this book is available from the British Library.

For a full list of Atlases in the series, plus forthcoming titles and details of
our surgical, dental and veterinary Atlases, please write to Wolfe Medical
Publications Ltd, 2-16 Torrington Place, London WC1E 7LT

Introduction

A deliberate attempt has been made to concentrate on those gynaecological conditions which are visible on inspection, with or without the aid of a speculum or colposcope. This means that lesions of the uterus, ovaries and fallopian tubes are largely neglected, even though they might be visualised with a laparoscope, or at laparotomy. It will be appreciated that a lot of common conditions as well as a few of the rare conditions which may be encountered in clinical practice are considered.

A diagnosis cannot be made without knowledge or experience. It is hoped that this atlas will help undergraduate and postgraduate students to gain this knowledge more quickly. The principle symptoms of a condition are given whenever appropriate so that the full benefits of this type of book can be gained. The treatment of those illustrated conditions principally related to parts of the genital tract which can be inspected, will also be given. The reader should be aware that this will inevitably result in a bias towards surgery. This is contrary to everyday clinical gynaecological practice, since for every woman attending with symptoms, only one out of every four or five requires an operation.

The most important aid to diagnosis is the information gained from taking a careful history from the patient or her relatives. In gynaecology, this is of particular significance since the diagnosis can usually be limited to two or three possibilities before any examination is performed. The number of possibilities is reduced still further after a full general examination, and in particular the examination of the breasts and abdomen. In many cases, the least important part of the gynaecologist's examination is the pelvic examination. This is because it will usually confirm a diagnosis already made from the history and symptoms. It should, however, always be included providing that it is possible to perform.

A rectal examination is useful either when a vaginal examination is not allowed on religious grounds, or in the investigation of children or babies. It also has a special role in the assessment of pelvic malignancy or when pathology of the Pouch of Douglas or uterosacral ligaments is suspected.

The additional help that can be obtained with a colposcope for assessing lesions of the vulva, vagina and cervix should not be underestimated. Unfortunately, whilst it is not routinely used, it is hoped that the reader will gain some idea of the help that one can obtain by using it, if it is available.

Contents

Acknowledgements

It would have been impossible to produce this Atlas without the help of colleagues in the Department of Obstetrics and Gynaecology. My predecessor, Professor W.I.C. Morris, left an excellent selection of slides of both common and rare conditions, collected whilst he held the Chair of Obstetrics and Gynaecology in Manchester University from 1949 to 1972. Another valuable source of material came from the Department of Medical Illustration, at Manchester Royal Infirmary, who have, over the years, built up a large collection of teaching slides. Additional material has been obtained from Dr P. Donnai, Professor M. Elstein and Mr P.C. Steptoe. The ultrasonic material has been kindly provided by Dr Valerie Jones and Dr Maureen Gowland. The colposcopy section for this book has been provided and written by Dr E. Blanche Butler, Senior Lecturer in Cytopathology, from her personal collection of cases as a consequence of the excellent service she provides for Gynaecologists in the North Western Region. I should also like to thank my secretary, Mrs Pauline Morris, for her invaluable help whilst having so many other tasks to perform. Finally, I should like to thank my wife for her personal sacrifices of time and leisure during the preparation of this Atlas.

Examination of the gynaecological patient

General examination

A full general examination is an essential part of every gynaecological examination. The general appearance and manner of the patient should be noted. Evidence of anaemia, wasting or hirsutism are fairly obvious. The neck should be examined, which should include palpation of the thyroid gland and supraclavicular fossa, for lymph nodes. Examination of the heart and lungs should be carried out after inspection of the breasts. The blood pressure should be taken and then any blood samples which may be considered relevant. Palpation of the breasts should always be carried out in order to exclude any abnormal masses.

Abdominal examination

An abdominal examination should always be carried out before pelvic or rectal examinations. The usual order is: inspection, palpation and percussion. The latter is often neglected, but is essential in helping to diagnose a tumour or the presence of free fluid (ascites) in the abdomen. All tumours arising from the pelvic organs are dull to percussion unless a loop of bowel is adherent and in front of it. It is important to remember that the bladder should always be emptied prior to any examination because it is the commonest physiological lower abdominal swelling encountered, followed by the physiological enlargement of the uterus during pregnancy. The kidneys, liver and spleen should be routinely palpated to exclude pathological conditions which may produce gynaecological symptoms, or, alternatively, influence the management of the patient. Although not strictly abdominal the area below the inguinal ligaments must be palpated to check for the presence or absence of lymph nodes or hernia. Since most gynaecologists also practice obstetrics, they should be particularly competent at abdominal palpation and pelvic examination because of the acquired skill gained by examining women in the ante natal period and during labour.

Generally, the flatter the hand is held, the lighter the palpation, the more the information gained. Warm hands help the examiner and are preferable for the patient.

The pelvic examination

Before examining a patient it is essential to have a good light and a suitable couch. The standard medical couch is suitable, although many prefer a shorter couch with foot rests. The latter is not in general use in the United Kingdom except for colposcopy examinations. The patient's bladder should be empty just as for any abdominal examination. A loaded rectum may interfere with a proper pelvic assessment and the findings might then have to be re-assessed when the bowel has been emptied. It is usual and preferable for doctors (especially male doctors) to have a nurse or chaperone present during the examination. The patient should always be covered up as much as possible in order to avoid embarrassment during the examination. This is particularly important in the teaching situation when undergraduates or postgraduates are present. Each part of the genital tract should be examined in a logical sequence: vulva, vagina, cervix, body of the uterus, ovaries or appendages (the fallopian tubes are not normally palpable), the uterosacral ligaments and Pouch of Douglas.

It is preferable to use sterile disposable gloves and autoclaved instruments in order to avoid transmitting infections, particularly trichomonas and monilial infections, from one woman to another. A non-greasy lubricant is preferable to both patient and examiner for application to speculum and gloves. All lubricant or discharge should be wiped away with cotton wool or gauze when the pelvic examination has been completed.

There are several positions which may be used for carrying out a pelvic examination. Each has its merits and all are likely to be used at one time or another depending upon the diagnosis being considered.

The dorsal position, is the one most commonly used; the patient's knees are bent and allowed to fall apart. The patient will feel less exposed if her thighs and knees are partially covered. Although this position is ideal for inspection of the vulva and for bimanual palpation of the uterus and appendages, it is not as good as the lateral position for inspection of the vaginal walls and cervix, or for the demonstration of prolapse of the genital tract. If the patient is placed upon a short couch with foot rests the gynaecologist can sit or stand directly in front of the patient; otherwise the examiner should stand on the right side of the patient. The modified dorsal position is one in which the hand is inserted below the flexed thigh and is a position best combined with the left lateral position. The speculum examination is performed in the left lateral position. The bimanual examination is commenced in the same position the patient (remaining covered) then rotates to the modified dorsal position without the bimanual examination being interrupted.

The left lateral position is the most common lateral position: the patient lies on her left side with her arms in front of her and this enables a good inspection of the anus, perineum and the posterior parts of the vulva, vagina and cervix. It is the best position for demonstrating prolapse, stress incontinence and for minor operations on the cervix in the non-anaesthetised woman. A bimanual examination is not as satisfactory as in the dorsal position unless it is associated with the modified dorsal position.

The semi-prone position of Sims is one in which the left arm is placed behind the patient's back. This position with the use of a Sim's speculum is ideal for the inspection of the anterior vaginal wall and cervix because when the introitus is opened the vagina fills out with air. It is also the least embarrassing position for the patient but it was devised by Sims for operating on vesico-vaginal fistulas. However, the patient's abdomen is not readily accessible and movement by the patient is limited due to the positioning of her arm.

The full lithotomy position, is usually used for operations or for examination under anaesthesia. The thighs are more flexed than would be obtained by the use of a short couch with foot supports. The knee-chest position is rarely used except for certain operations: e.g. insertion of radium; culdoscopy; or repair of vesico-vaginal fistula. It is not liked by patients who find it both embarrassing and inelegant.

Whatever the position used, inspection should precede palpation. An inspection of the vulva, vagina and cervix should include tests for prolapse; a cervical smear; and high vaginal swabs for culture. Speculum examination of the vagina and cervix normally precedes a bimanual vaginal examination. The principle disadvantage is: it is not easy to choose the appropriate size of speculum until palpation estimates the size of the vagina. This difficulty can be surmounted by careful attention to the patient's medical history: whether or not

that patient has had any previous examinations; previous pregnancies; has coitus or uses tampons; and, on inspection, a careful appraisal of the introitus. If a patient is a virgin the opening of the hymen may be sufficient to allow a one finger examination or the passage of a narrow speculum without discomfort, especially if the patient uses tampons during menstruation. If a tentative approach makes it clear that an examination is unlikely and also that sufficient information cannot be obtained from a rectal examination, then examination under anaesthesia is indicated.

The advantage of passing a speculum first is that any vaginal discharge can be seen and specimens of it taken. The epithelium of the cervix is undisturbed and satisfactory material for cytological examination can be obtained from the cervix or posterior fornix. Some lesions of the vagina and cervix bleed when touched and if this occurred initially with a bimanual examination, then a subsequent inspection would be difficult and cytological assessment impossible.

In passing a speculum it should be remembered that both the Sim's and bivalve speculum are designed for direct application. They should not be inserted with their blade in line with the cleft of the vulva and then rotated in the vagina. The vagina is wider from side to side than from front to back. Initially only one finger should be inserted for a bimanual palpation. The second finger should be inserted only when the muscles around the vagina are relaxed and when it is obvious that a two finger examination can be carried out without causing pain. In any type of vaginal examination it is important to remember that the direction of the vagina is upwards and backwards.

The beginner is often surprised to learn that the palpation of the pelvic organs is done predominantly by the abdominal hand rather than the finger(s) inserted into the vagina. In order to feel the uterus the cervix is pushed backwards, thus rotating the body of the uterus downwards and forwards. The abdominal hand, which should be placed at the umbilical level, is then gradually moved downwards towards the suprapubic region until the uterus is caught and pressed against the fingers in the anterior fornix. If the uterus cannot be felt, it is therefore lying above and behind the abdominal hand. The expert can usually deduce the position of the uterus from the position of the cervix: for example, if the cervix points to the sacrum and coccyx the uterus is anteverted, but points to the pubic symphysis if the uterus is retroverted. It is also essential to remember that a gentle one-finger bimanual examination will always reveal more information than a painful two-finger examination. If the patient does tense her abdominal and pelvic floor muscles in the dorsal position, then the most effective method of overcoming this, is for the patient to arch her back and support herself on her shoulders and feet. She should do this unaided, lifting her buttocks two or three inches off the couch. The powerful extensor muscles of the back are required for this manoeuvre and thus ensure complete relaxation of the flexor muscles of the abdomen. If, in this manoeuvre, the patient's thighs are also adducted, by making sure the patient keeps her knees far apart, the pelvic floor muscles also relax. This is simpler and more effective than asking the patient to breath deeply in the hope that sufficient relaxation will be gained upon breathing out.

In a bimanual examination one should determine the size, shape, position, mobility and consistency of the uterus, and also notice any tenderness on movement or palpation of the uterus. The normal uterus is tender when squeezed between two hands. Since the position and direction of the cervix are guides to the position of the uterus, the speculum inspection of the cervix usually indicates whether or not the uterus is anteverted or retroverted. Normal fallopian tubes are never palpable, even in the anaesthetised patient. Palpation of the ovaries is more difficult, for they, like testicles, produce slight discomfort. They are more laterally placed than is usually appreciated by the beginner. The vaginal fingers are inserted in the lateral fornix and the abdominal hand brought down towards the anterior iliac spine and then in-wards to the mid-inguinal point. If the vaginal fingers are pushing structures up into the lateral fornix, the ovary will usually be felt between the abdominal hand and vaginal fingers. If they are not felt, then the gynaecologist can be reasonably certain they are not enlarged. For those who use their right hand for examination, the right ovary is often more palpable than the left. Nowadays, the policy of using the left hand to feel the left appendage is not common practice; most gynae-cologists are trained to use one hand only.

The usual tests carried out during a pelvic examination, namely a vaginal swab and cervical smear, have been referred to briefly earlier. The vaginal swab is usually taken from the posterior fornix of the vagina (high vaginal swab) and especially at the site of discharge. The cervical smear should be taken using a wooden spatula and rotated through 360° at the external cervical os. Vulval swabs should be taken if vulvitis is present or if the patient complains of pruritus vulvae. Cervical and urethral swabs are taken when gonococcal infection is suspected. In all cases, swabs should be cultured immediately, though this is not always practically possible. Special transport-ing media have therefore been devised in which the swabs can be inserted into directly. For example, Stuart's media is suitable for suspected gonococcal infections, whilst the Feinberg Whittington media are suitable for trichomonas vaginalis and monilial infections.

1 Ovarian cyst. Inspection of the abdomen reveals an abdominal swelling arising from the pelvis. In this case it was due to an ovarian cyst. The principle differential diagnoses include a full bladder, enlarged uterus due to pregnancy, fibroids, or other causes.

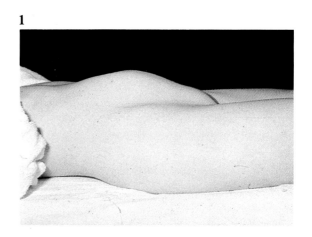

2 An enlarged abdomen due to pregnancy. The striae gravidarum can be seen above and below the umbilicus. Also visible is the mark left by a fetal stethoscope indicating the presence of some excess fluid in the skin. This patient had mild pre-eclampsia with oedema and hypertension.

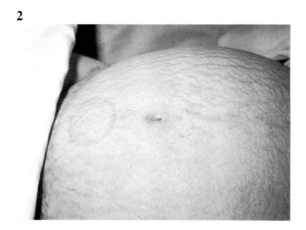

3 Malignant ovarian cyst and ascites. The patient has a large abdomen and is sitting up. The umbilicus is everted and a few veins are visible on the right side of the abdomen. The supraclavicular nodes were enlarged and are just visible in the left supraclavicular region.

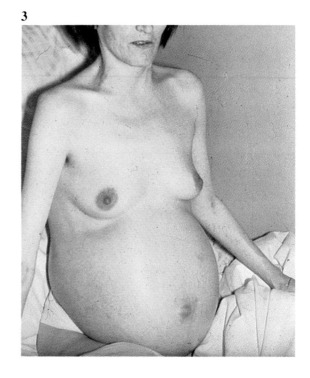

4 Breast changes in pregnancy. The breast is enlarged and its increased vascularity is demonstrated by the prominent veins. The pigmented area around the nipple is surrounded by Montgomery's tubules (the sebaceous glands in the areola of the breast, which becomes more prominent in pregnancy).

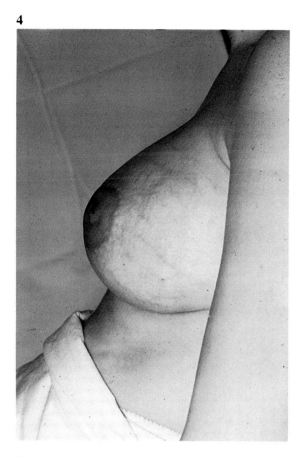

5 Inspection of the vulval area in the dorsal position. The amount of hair is variable and in the reproductive era, as in this case, it often obscures the labia and introitus.

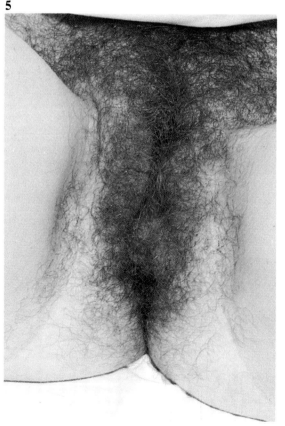

6 **Separation of the labia minora**, however, allows inspection of the introitus prior to the insertion of a lubricated specimen.

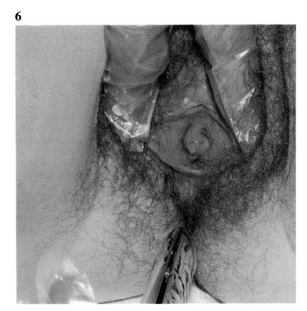

7 **The bivalve speculum is in position** but not yet opened. The handle of the speculum can be placed upwards (as in this case) or downwards to the anus. It is a matter of individual preference.

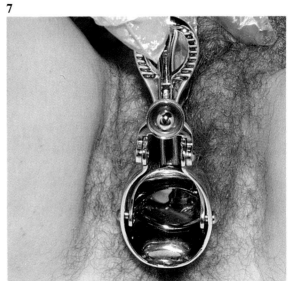

8 **The bivalve speculum is opened and locked.** The normal cervix and cervical os is exposed and visible. A cervical smear can be easily taken.

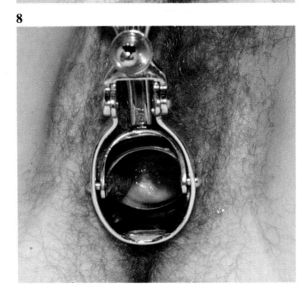

9 **The wooden cervical spatula in position** shown in a closer view. In order to take a satisfactory smear it should be rotated through 360°. The superficial cells which are obtained on the spatula are spread onto a clean glass slide and fixed immediately.

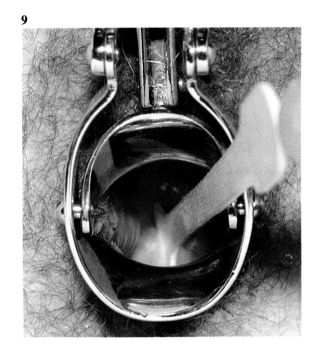

10 **Another type of bivalve speculum** in which the lock is placed at the side. A clear view of the cervix and the posterior fornix is obtained, but the anterior and posterior walls are obscured by the speculum blades.

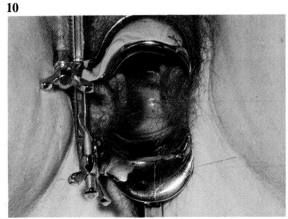

11 **A plastic circular speculum and plastic spatula.** A good exposure of the cervix. The vaginal walls can be seen only when the speculum is slowly removed.

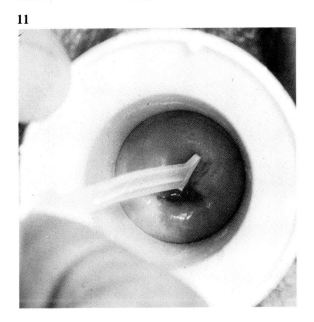

12 Prolapse. On coughing the prolapse appeared outside the vaginal orifice. The cervix and a cystocele are visible. All that one can determine on inspection is that the patient has, at least, a second degree uterine prolapse and cystocele. It is impossible to say whether there is an associated rectocele or enterocele.

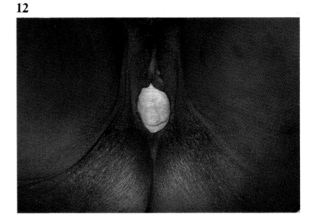

13 Inspection of the introitus in the lateral position. In order to obtain a good view of the introitus in either the Sims or the left lateral position, the buttock and the upper labia have to be elevated.

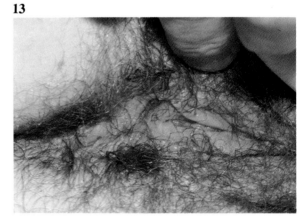

14 A bivalve speculum inserted in the lateral position. The left lateral wall is visible.

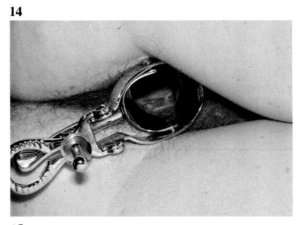

15 Left lateral position. A Sims' speculum has been inserted. With the buttocks held up there is a good exposure of the anterior vaginal wall and cervix. In this case a cervical smear is being taken.

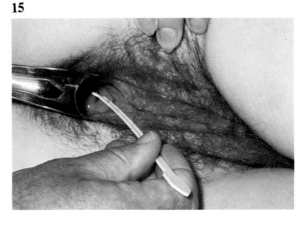

16 Bimanual examination in the dorsal position.
The fingers in the vagina steady the pelvic organs
and the structures palpable in the midline are felt
between the abdominal hand and the vaginal
fingers.

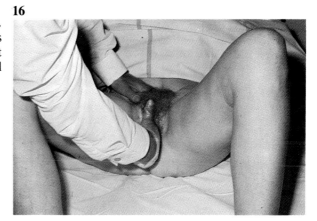

17 Palpation of the right ovary. The vaginal
fingers are placed in the right lateral fornix and the
abdominal hand moves down the right iliac fossa
from the level of the iliac crest, towards and then
below the mid-inguinal point.

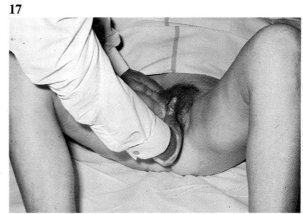

18 Palpation of the left ovary. The modern
practice is to use the same hand in the vagina
rather than to change hands. The abdominal hand
moves down the left iliac fossa from the level of the
iliac crest, towards and then below, the mid-
inguinal point.

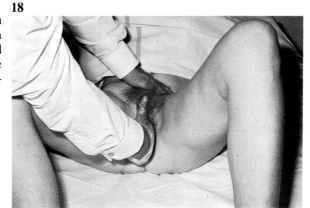

The vulva

The skin of the vulva is subject to the same disease processes which can occur in any hair bearing skin area on the body. Those described here are only a few of the more common ones encountered, although other types are also depicted.

Infection around the apertures of hair follicles is often caused by organisms, particularly *staphylococcus aureus*, present on the skin following mild trauma such as scratching. This may lead to folliculitis, but deeper infection of the skin can lead to boils and carbuncles, which may be recurrent. Contributory factors are: the irritation of tight underclothing; the wearing of sanitary pads; lack of cleanliness; diabetes; and a lowered general resistance. Single abscesses, often representing infection of a retention cyst of an apocrine or sebaceous gland, have the same clinical characteristics of a boil and are treated in the same way.

When the vulval epithelium is thin and inactive, as in the pre-menstrual and post-menstrual phases of a woman's life, any of the organisms to which it is normally resistant can set up a simple vulvitis. In these age groups, it can be associated with fusion of the labia. This type of vulvitis is often associated with vaginitis.

Herpes genitalis in women takes the form of multiple, shallow ulcers with red margins and these are found on the labia and around the introitus. Symptoms are limited to pain and local pruritus.

Intertrigo can occur and is a superficial inflammation of the external genitalia. It is often caused by chafing, especially in obese women during hot weather. The presence of a persistent vaginal discharge will prolong the irritation.

Tinea cruris – a fungal infection or ringworm of the groin – may be found. Other sources of fungal infection such as hands or feet are more common with secondary involvement of the vulval region.

Psoriasis of the vulva is not uncommon and the presenting complaint may be pruritus. It is usually part of a generalised psoriasis and the lesions are similar in appearance.

Varicose veins of the vulva occur most often during pregnancy or as a result of high parity. They are usually associated with varicose veins of the lower limbs. Oedema of the vulva may occur with local infections or with chronic conditions of the kidneys or heart because of the loose texture of the subcutaneous labial tissue. The term elephantiasis is applied to chronic hypertrophic tissue changes secondary to excessive lymph stasis. In the tropics, the commonest cause of elephantiasis is the parasitic worm, *Wuchereria bancrofti*. Obstruction of the lymphatics which drain the vulva may occur as the end result of chronic conditions such as tuberculosis, lymphogranuloma inguinale and other sexually transmitted diseases and are more common in temperate zones.

A haematoma of the vulva may be secondary to a fall, a blow, surgical trauma or rupture of a varix. The blood is slowly absorbed even from minor extravasations. A large collection of blood may distend the labia and spread into the ischiorectal fossa and buttock.

Pruritus vulvae is common in diabetic women. Indeed, glycosuria, whether due to diabetes or not, is often associated with a diffuse inflammation. In most cases, the vulvitis (vulvovaginitis) is the result of a superimposed monilial infection. The growth of various fungi is encouraged by the presence of carbohydrates which the vulva is contaminated with under these circumstances. As a result irritation, excoriation and furuncles are common complications.

In the acute stage of *Trichomonas vaginalis* infection a vulvitis is usually present with congestion of the vestibule and the inner aspects of the labia minora.

The symptoms of acute gonorrhoea of the vulva, which may appear one to several days after contact, are often mild and overlooked. The patient may experience burning on micturition, leucorrhoea and itching in the region of the vestibule. Often the principle symptoms, if they occur, are after the next menstrual period when the ascending infection has resulted in an acute salpingitis. Chronic foci of infection may persist in the peri-urethral tubules, endocervix, Bartholin's gland and rectum.

In acute Bartholinitis the opening of the ducts, normally inconspicuous, become apparent because of the surrounding inflammation. Although the infection can resolve completely, it usually remains and a resulting abscess forms which ultimately drains through the lower vaginal wall. Chronic infection results in the gland which becomes permanently enlarged and fibrotic so that it can be felt between the fingers like a small hard pea. Many Bartholin's abscesses are secondarily infected cysts.

The sexually transmitted diseases affect the vulva as well as other parts of the genital tract. The initial symptoms are often overlooked, and the later effects of the disease processes are more often noted.

All cysts and benign tumours of the vulva usually cause the patient to complain of a swelling or lump, but they may also be noticed as incidental findings. The causes are many and varied, and include some of the conditions already mentioned, which may present with pruritus as the predominant symptom.

There are also vaginal, cervical and uterine tumours which may project through the introitus. Finally, one should not forget the malignant conditions which include the commoner squamous cell carcinoma, or occasional adenocarcinomas, sarcomas, and melanoma as primary tumours. Secondary malignant tumours, including choriocarcinoma and lymphoma, may be blood borne from any site.

The vulval skin is commonly the site of chronic and persistent changes, all of which lead to considerable variation in terminology. Whilst most of the changes are benign, a small proportion of the women with these chronic changes will progress over a number of years to develop a carcinoma *in situ*, or will actually develop invasive carcinoma. Providing this possibility is borne in mind the terminology is perhaps less important. The chronic vulval epithelial dystrophies are sometimes called leucoplakia, lichen sclerosis, kraurosis vulvae and senile atrophy. The two principle views regarding the aetiology of chronic vulval dystrophies are either: (i) they are manifestations of the same pathological process, or, (ii) they represent separate and distinct processes.

Principle modes of involvement of the vulva in producing gynaecological symptoms	
Infections	– acute vulvitis, furuncle or carbuncle, warts (condylomata accumata), tuberculosis, syphilis.
Injury	– haematoma.
Vascular	– varicose veins, oedema.
Lymphatic	– elephantiasis.
Congenital abnormalities	– enlarged clitoris, hypertrophy of one or both labia minora, phimosis of the glans clitoris (secretion of smegma will also cause a swelling).
Retention cysts	– Sebaceous cyst, inclusion dermoid, remnants of the Wolffian duct system.
Endometriosis	– cysts or deposits.
Benign tumours	– papilloma, fibromyoma, neuroma, neurofibroma, lipoma, angioma, hydroblastoma, sweat gland tumour (hidradenoma).
Malignant tumours	– Primary (or secondary) carcinoma, sarcoma, melanoma.
Bartholin's gland	– Bartholin's abscess, cyst or infection, adenoma, adenocarcinoma.
Urethral conditions	– prolapse of urethra, caruncle, carcinoma, cyst of Skene's tubule, diverticulum of the urethra.
Hernia	– inguinal hernia, hydrocele of the canal of Nuck, varicocele of the round ligament, tumours of the round ligament. Prolapse – vaginal and/or uterine, inversion of the uterus.

19 Variation in the size of labia minora. The labia are drawn out sideways. The clitoral hood is also apparent with the clitoris visible between the two folds.

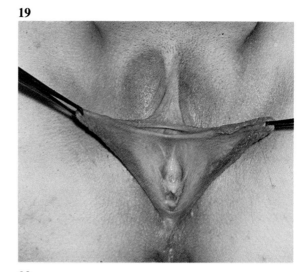

20 A lateral view of the labia minora shown in **19**. They are relatively thin and long.

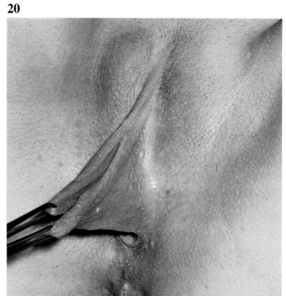

21 Imperforate hymen. Below the urethra there is a membrane with bluish discolouration. The labia minora are normal in appearance compared with **19** and **20**. The variation in the clitoral hood can also be noticed.

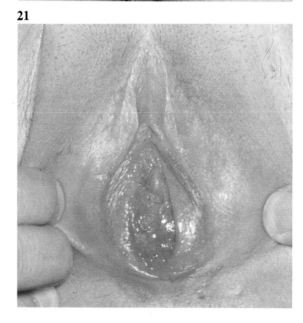

22 Imperforate hymen. Greater distension of the collected menstrual blood in the vagina. The labia are slightly darker and more marked than in the previous example (**20**) but are within normal limits.

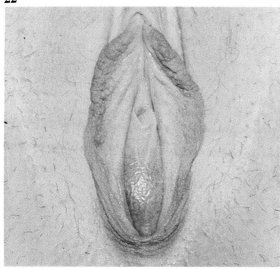

23 Imperforate hymen. Note the more obvious distention of the membrane when the labia minora are separated.

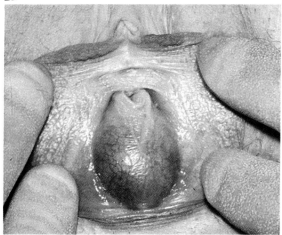

24 Incised imperforate hymen showing the menstrual blood which had collected behind the membrane, pouring out immediately after incision.

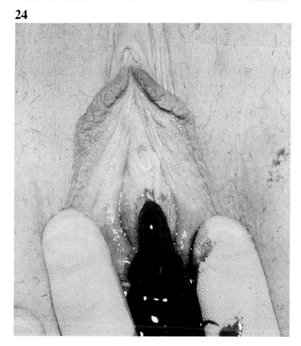

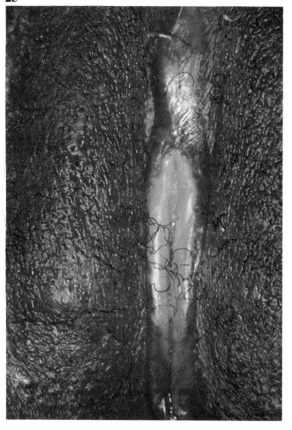

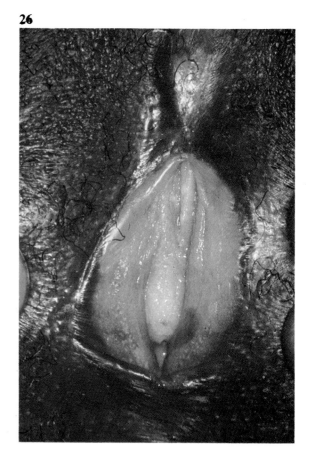

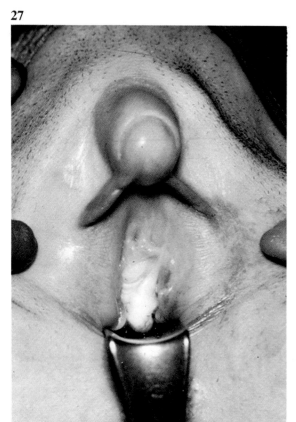

25 Female circumcision. The crura of the clitoris has been almost completely removed by circumcision. Only scar tissue is visible.

26 Female circumcision. Opening the vaginal introitus shows the absence of the clitoral hood and clitoris. The labia minora are united below the site of the circumcision, but above the urethra.

27 An enlarged clitoris as a result of virilisation. This may occur with the adrenogenital syndrome, the rare arrhenoblastomas and drug therapy, especially androgens.

28

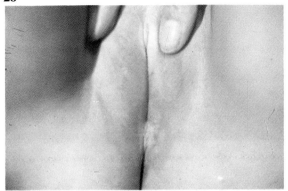

29

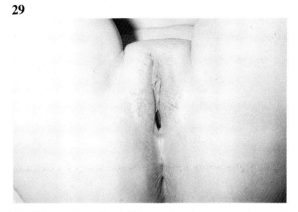

28 The vulva of a young girl age 10 complaining of pruritus vulvae. There are predominantly red areas with white patches in the region of the clitoris and perineal area. Biopsy revealed changes similar to lichen sclerosis in a post-menopausal woman. Symptomatic relief was gained by local hydrocortisone. Awaiting menarche in the hope that the condition will improve spontaneously before any oestrogen therapy is considered.

29 The vulva of a child, age 6, who complained of pruritus vulvae. Minimal changes to be noted, except a little cracking of perineum. The diagnosis was made by the nursing staff who found thread worms on routine testing for these when the child was an in-patient.

30

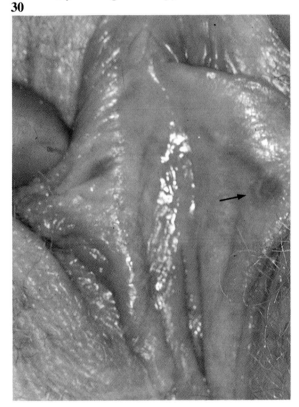

31

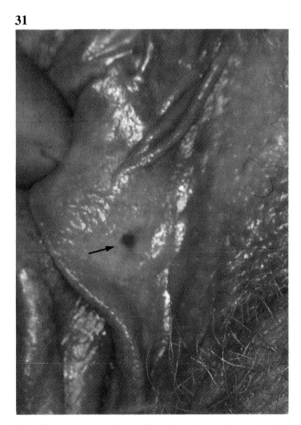

30 Ulcer of labia minora considered to be due to herpes infection. It was noted when the patient complained of pruritus vulvae. The patient also had marked oral herpes infection.

31 Posterior surface of labia minora shown in **30**. This shows the inflammatory reaction at the base of the ulcer.

32

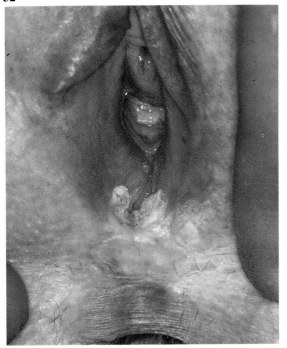

33

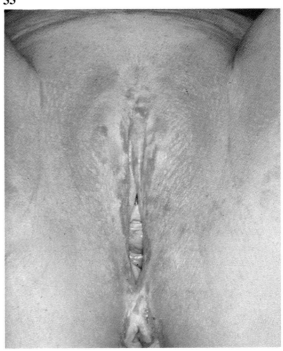

32 Pruritus vulvae. A definite white patch (leucoplakia) is visible at the posterior part of the introitus. The patient was postmenopausal and no other abnormality was found.

33 Chronic monilial vulvitis. Note the healed areas and appearance of the skin as well as the ulcerated and raw areas.

34

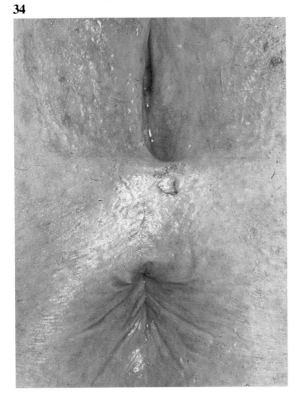

34 Peri-anal monilial infection. A small area of trauma caused by scratching is present near the vaginal orifice.

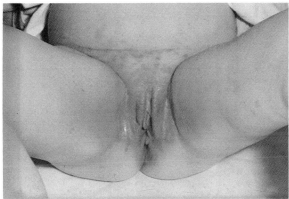

35 **Monilial vulvovaginitis** in a diabetic patient.

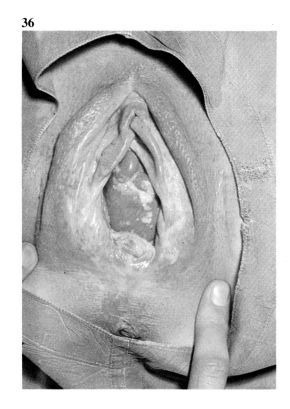

36 **Monilial vulvovaginitis.** The typical plaques of monilial discharge are seen on the anterior vaginal wall.

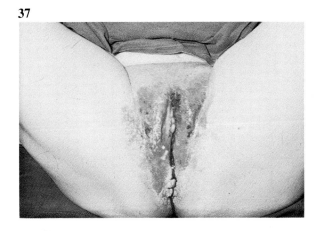

37 **Severe vulvovaginitis.** The patient had been using talc to ease her symptoms of pruritus. She was prepared for multiple biopsies to exclude malignancy. The biopsies were negative. Note the bleeding from the raw areas.

38 **Hidradenoma.** The patient presented with a traumatised area on the vulva from scratching as a result of pruritus vulvae. Biopsy of the ulcerated area revealed the lesion to be a hidradenoma and was later removed by excision. These lesions, when ulcerated, can mimic a carcinoma.

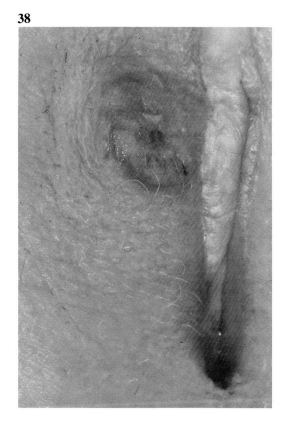

39 **Acute vulvitis** with oedema of labia minora and clitoris.

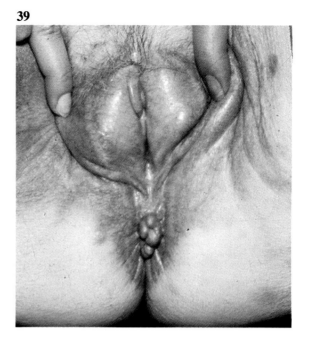

40 **Pruritus vulvae** was suffered by this obese patient for 20 years. She was noted to have leucoplakia, and at the age of 61 had a local vulvectomy for leucoplakia. The histology revealed 'extensive leucoplakia with patchy areas of superficial ulceration. The epithelium showed marked thickening, hyperkeratinisation and hyperplasia with what appeared to be early carcinomatous changes in one area.'

The ensuing series of pictures are selected from a continuous follow-up over a period of a further 13 years. During which time, biopsies were carried out. The first shows the perineum when aged 66, i.e. five years after the local vulvectomy had been performed.

41 **Appearances of the vulva in the dorsal position.** Five and a half years after local vulvectomy. The groin, mons pubis and upper part of the introitus are shown for comparison with the view shown in **40** although there is a time interval.

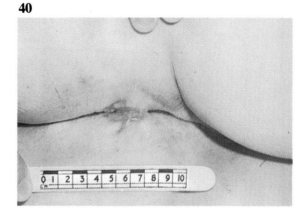

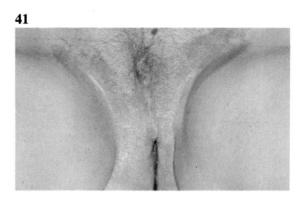

42 Seven years after the local vulvectomy. Symptoms were relieved by local application of hydrocortisone and hibitane creams.

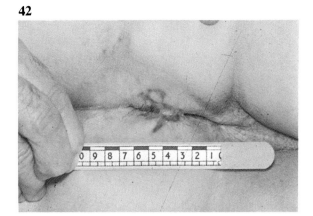

43 Ten years after vulvectomy (aged 71). This picture was taken four months after local excision of a raised thickened area on the anterior part of the vulva had been carried out. It was histologically proved to be a keratinising squamous cell carcinoma of the vulva.

The adjacent epithelium showed acanthosis and hyperplasia (leucoplakia).

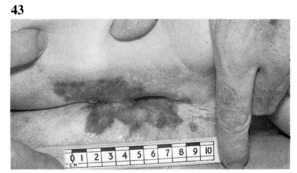

44 Appearance in the dorsal position twelve and a half years after a local vulvectomy for leucoplakia and symptoms of pruritus vulvae on and off over a period of 20 years.

45 Thirteen years after local vulvectomy and subsequent local excision of a nodule which had undergone carcinomatous change. Symptoms of pruritus relieved by local steroid creams. No clinical evidence of recurrence. The patient's general condition remained reasonable despite hypertension.

The patient died shortly before her 75th birthday from a cerebral vascular accident.

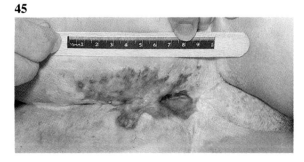

46 A multifocal microinvasive basal cell carcinoma was revealed at biopsy. She had complained of pruritus vulvae and had abnormal vulval cytology. A vulvectomy was performed.

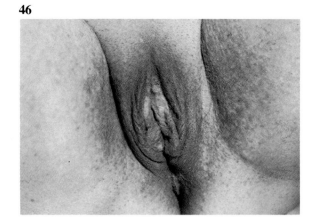

47 Complaint of pruritus vulvae plus the presence of a sore. The clinical features are suggestive of an early carcinoma. Smears and biopsy of the lesion only revealed an *in situ* lesion. She had a radical vulvectomy. The inguinal nodes were normal and the final diagnosis was carcinoma *in situ*.

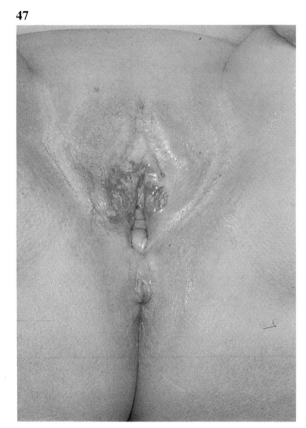

48 Leucoplakia clinically. There is considerable variation between the appearance in the groin and around the labia minora. There was no evidence of carcinoma on biopsy. Symptoms were relieved by local hydrocortisone cream.

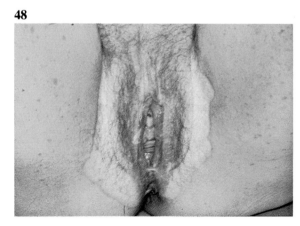

49

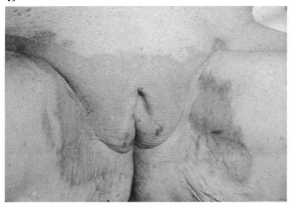

50

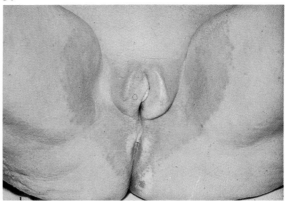

49   Alteration in pigmentation of vulval region as a result of chronic skin changes associated with poor hygiene, obesity and chafing.

50   Skin changes in the groins. The vulva, the site of monilial infection, and symptoms of pruritus vulvae.

51

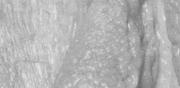

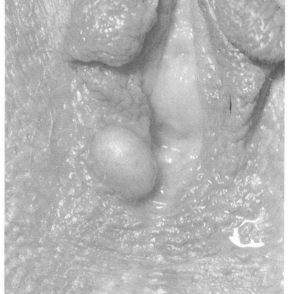

51   Sebaceous cyst of the vulva. A small lump was noticed, otherwise symptomless. The treatment is as for sebaceous cysts elsewhere, namely removal by excision.

52

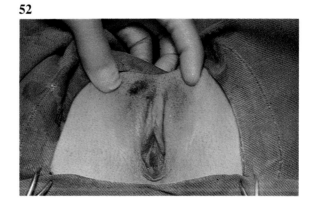

52   A papilloma on the upper part of the right labia majora which had bled slightly on shaving. Although symptomless, its removal was requested by the patient. The principle reason for her operation was previous trauma to the vagina and introitus. The only visible sign being a contused area at the right side of the introitus.

53 Multiple melanoma of vulva. Pigmented and easily recognisable.

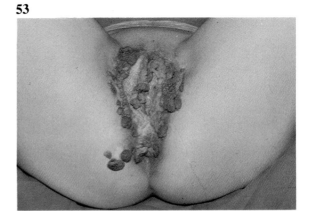

54 Sebaceous glands of labia with black domed secretion. Similar to Cock's peculiar tumour in which septic ulcerations of a neglected sebaceous cyst may simulate an epithelioma.

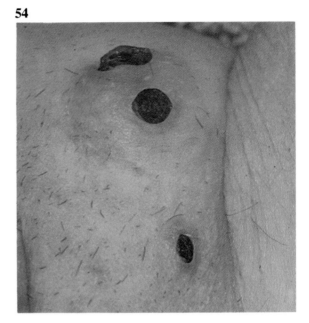

55 Fibroma of the vulva. Diagnosis was confirmed after excision.

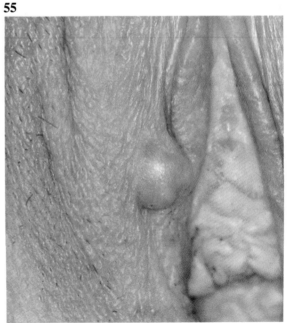

56

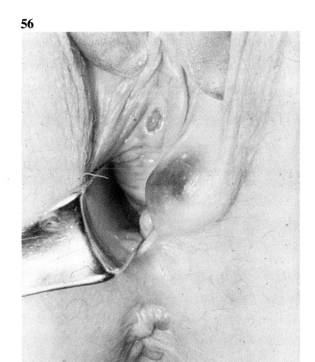

57

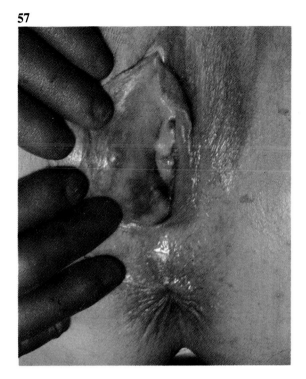

58

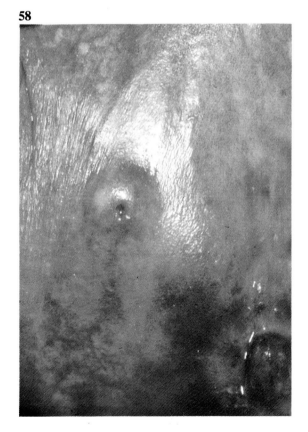

56 Endometriosis of vulva. The nodule gradually increased in size. The patient had extensive pelvic endometriosis treated by conservative surgery and a subsequent pseudo-pregnancy course of oestrogen and progestogen. This did not appear to influence the vulval lesion which was subsequently excised.

57 Endometriosis of the labia minora. A small nodule with a dimple on the right side.

58 A closer view of the endometriotic nodule shown in **57**. The small dimple filled up cyclically when ovulation was not being suppressed.

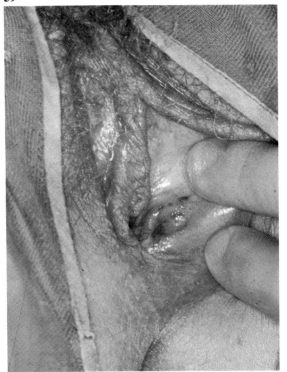

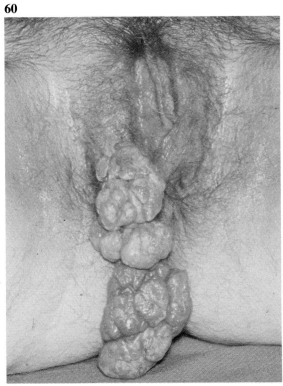

59 Endometriosis of the labia minora. An ulcerated lesion. Adjacent to the larger ulcer are additional smaller ones above and at each side.

60 A variety of condylomata arising from a wide base, which might be mistaken for pedunculated papilloma.

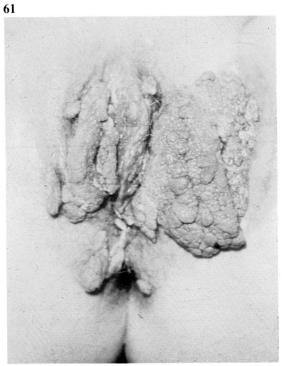

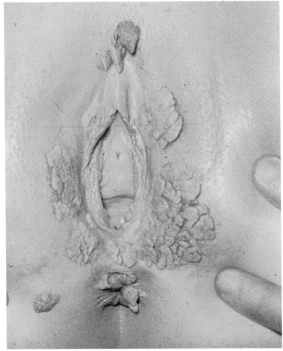

61 Condylomata acumata: a more typical appearance.

62 Condylomata. More discrete plaques involving vulva and anal areas. Whilst they may be treated with Podophyllin compound paint BPC as an outpatient, those with broad bases often have to be removed under anaesthesia.

63 Multiple condylomata involving, in particular, the lower part of the labia minora, perineum and the anal region.

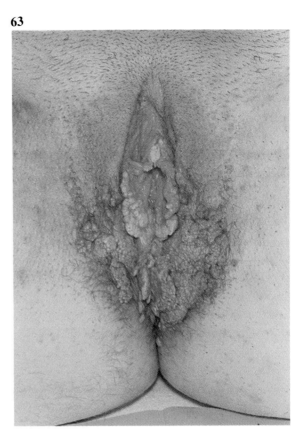

64 Multiple sebaceous cysts of the vulva.

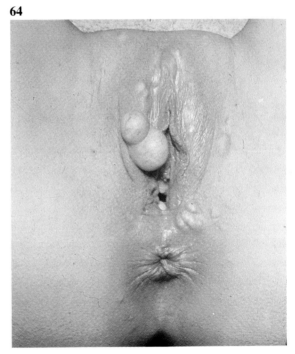

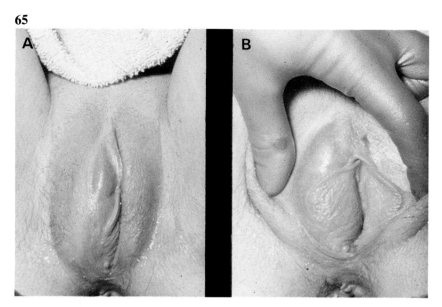

65 Bartholin's abscess. The cyst is less marked with the vulva in the normal position (A) than in (B) where the labia are separated. It is important to remember that they are usually multiloculated when incising an abscess to prevent recurrence. Marsupialisation is more effective.

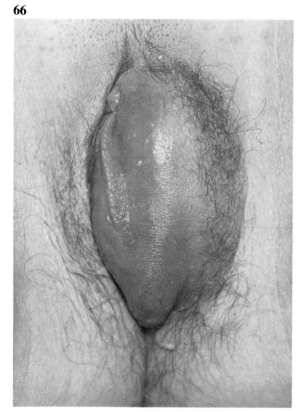

66 A large Bartholin's abscess of the left side obscuring the introitus.

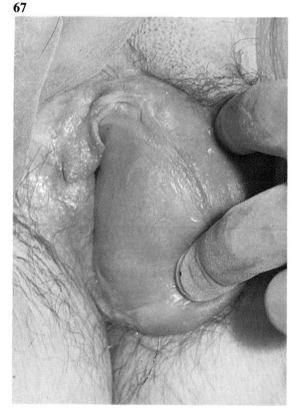

67 The acute Bartholin's abscess shown in **66**. There is oedema of the labia minora, and when it and the abscess are moved aside the introitus and right labia minora are exposed.

68

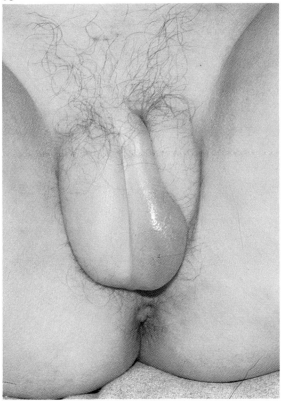

69

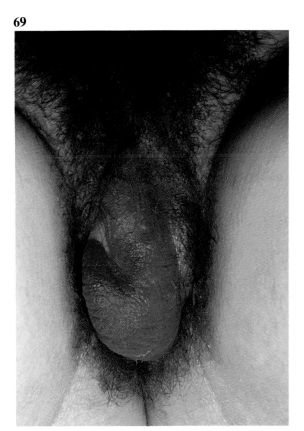

68 Oedema of the vulva secondary to the nephrotic syndrome.

69 Haematoma of the vulva can follow injury (as in this case) or trauma of childbirth.

70

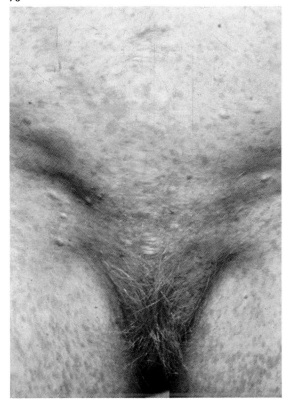

70 Multiple neurofibromatosis (von Recklinghausen's disease) involving the lower abdomen and groins. The lesions were symptomless in this patient but can undergo sarcomatous changes.

71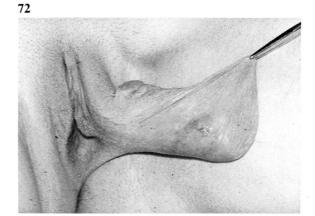

72

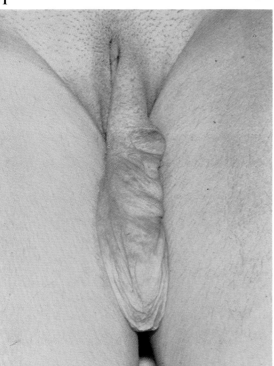

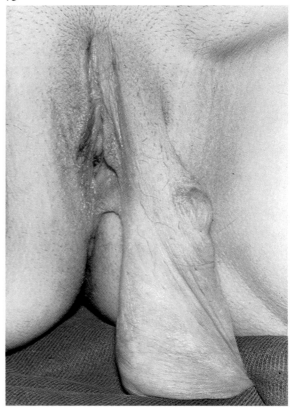

73

71   A pedunculated fibroma. The loose tissue surrounding it is somewhat similar in appearance to a scrotum.

72   The pedunculated fibroma drawn out sideways to reveal its broad base from the labia majora.

73   The patient's legs have been separated and the pedunculated swelling drawn out to reveal its full length.

74

74   A lipoma of the vulva arising from a broad base.

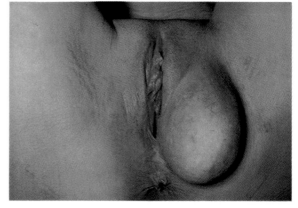

75 **A pedunculated lipoma** arising from the vulva. The treatment of lipoma and fibroma is surgical excision.

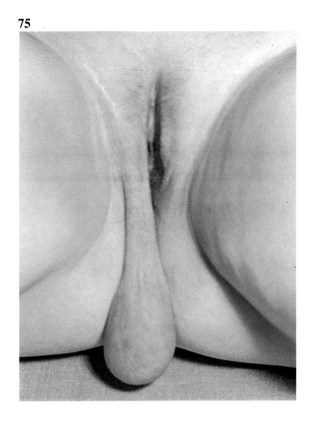

76 **A melanoma of the vulva** also involving the clitoral area. It was growing rapidly and bled on touching, but histologically the biopsy was indeterminate. Because of the possibility of malignancy a radical vulvectomy was performed. The final diagnosis was a benign lesion.

76

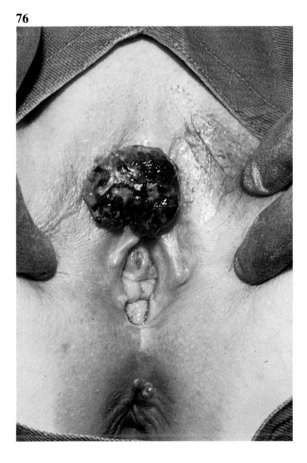

77 Metastatic vaccination. A young child transmitted it by scratching the site of the vaccination and her vulva.

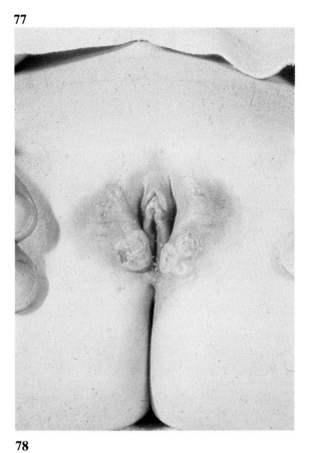

78 Elephantiasis. This is a late stage of filariasis as a consequence of the blockage of the lymphatics. It was due to the parasitic worm, *Wuchereria bancrofti* and transmitted by mosquitoes.

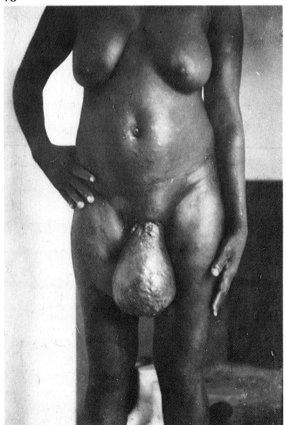

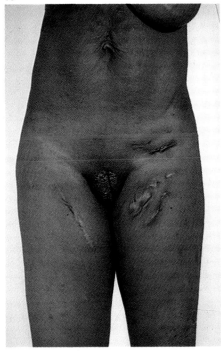

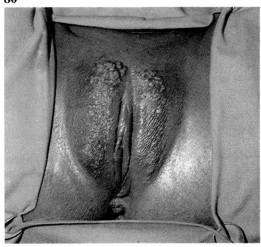

79 Lymphoedema of the vulva secondary to inguinal lymphatic sclerosis following tuberculous adenitis. The scars are a result of surgery for removal of the enlarged glands and the involvement of the skin by the tuberculous adenitis.

80 The vulva of the patient shown in **79**. There is some lymphoedema as a result of tuberculous adenitis.

81

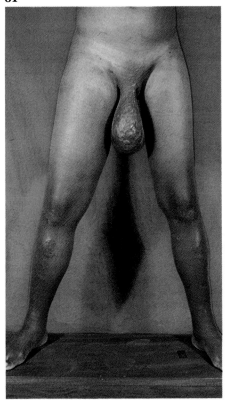

81 Lymphoedema of the right labia as a result of obstruction of the lymphatics. The right leg is also seen to be swollen when compared to the left. The left labia majora can be seen at the base of the swelling.

82 Melanoma of the vulva and abdominal wall.
It was rapidly growing and smears from the red
areas revealed malignant cells. Biopsy of several
areas revealed an *in situ*, possibly invasive, lesion.

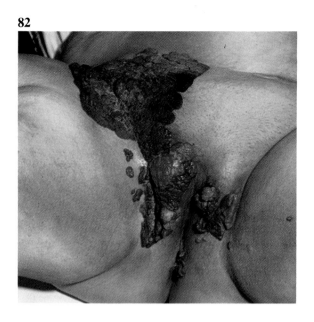

83 Melanoma of abdominal wall. This shows the
total area of abdominal involvement which is
incompletely shown in **82**. A radical vulvectomy
and excision of the whole abdominal area was
carried out. Histologically there was carcinoma *in
situ* only. This, and the patient's obesity, perhaps
explains why the patient was discharged home 24
days after the operation with the incisions
completely healed and covered.

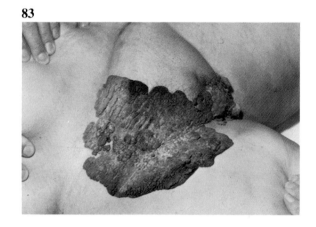

84 Melanoma of the vulva. This was a rapidly
growing tumour and histologically proved to be
malignant. The lesions contained pigmented, and
non-pigmented areas.

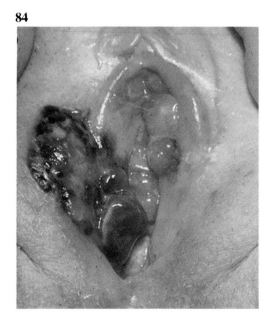

85

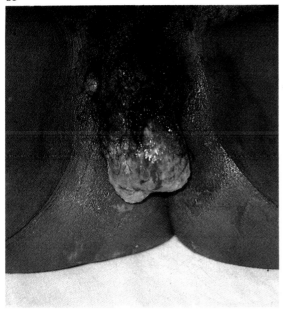

86

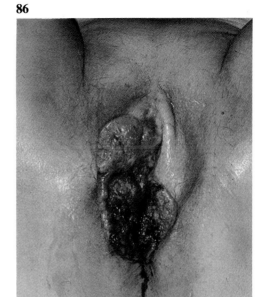

85 Carcinoma of the vulva. A large ulcerating mass with areas of necrotic tissue and superficial slough are visible. There are also streaks of blood over the tumour.

86 Carcinoma of the vulva. An ulcerating lesion of the right labia majora and minora. There is slight oedema of the left labia minora. The upper part of the tumour has not ulcerated.

87

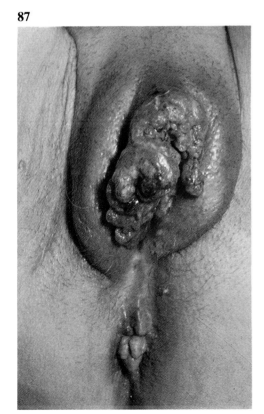

88

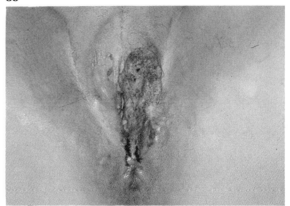

87 Carcinoma of the vulva. A cauliflower type of tumour involving the upper part of the vaginal introitus and clitoris.

88 Carcinoma of the vulva. An ulcerated carcinoma with a necrotic area in the centre. The cracking of the skin in the groins and on the mons pubis are the result of a long history of pruritus vulvae. The patient had, however, not sought medical advice about this symptom.

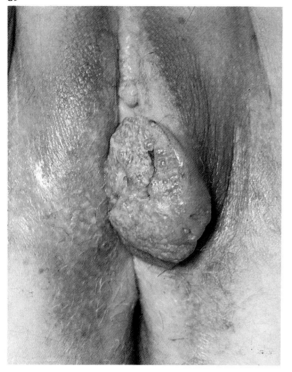

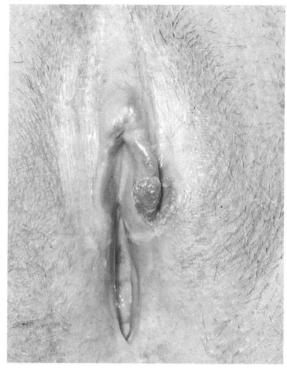

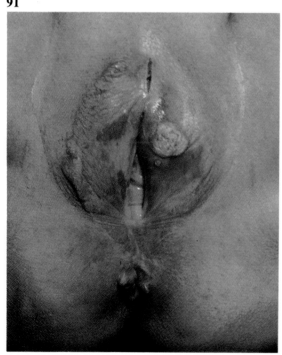

89 Vulval carcinoma. A polypoidal tumour of the left labia majora covering the introitus with a small nodule near the clitoris, which was also malignant. Despite its size, the inguinal and femoral nodes were free of tumour.

90 Vulval carcinoma. A small nodule of carcinoma at the lower part of the labia minora. Despite its size, the lymph nodes in the groins contained carcinoma in this case. The size of a tumour does not always reflect the extent of tumour spread.

91 Vulval carcinoma. A carcinoma with a small nodule below it, plus areas of leucoplakia.

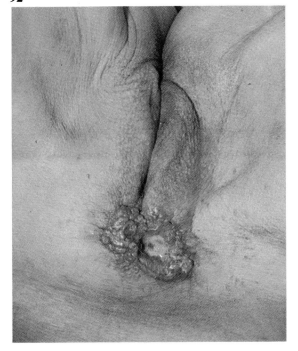

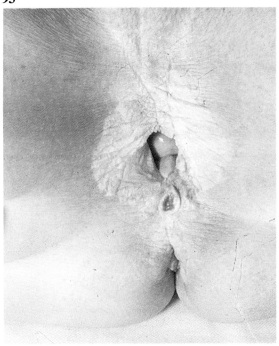

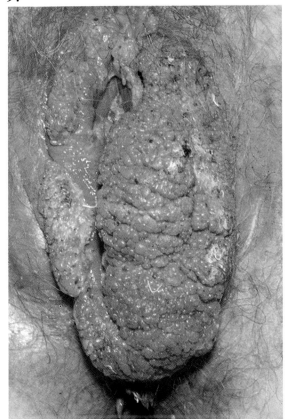

92　Anal carcinoma. The carcinoma involved the anus and part of the perineum. For complete cure it was considered necessary to excise the lower part of the rectum and for there to be a permanent colostomy.

93　Leucoplakia and local recurrence of carcinoma. This patient had previously had a local vulvectomy for leucoplakia. A small area of carcinoma found in the specimen was considered to have been completely excised and no further surgery was performed. The leukoplakia returned within five years and a year later there was this small ulcerated area in the perineum. This proved to be a squamous cell carcinoma.

94　Vulval carcinoma. A large carcinoma almost covering the whole of the introitus and labia minora. It is a proliferative mass.

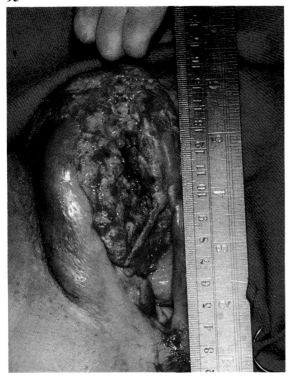

95 Vulval carcinoma. A large ulcerating mass involving the upper part of the labia, clitoral region and mons pubis.

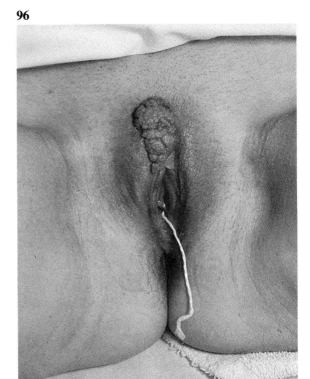

96 Vulval carcinoma. A carcinoma involving the clitoral region. The prognosis of a carcinoma in this position is generally worse because of the direct spread in the lymphatic connections beneath the symphysis pubis.

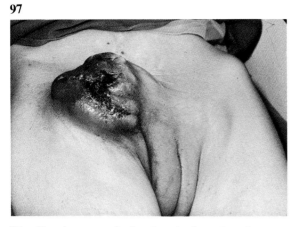

97 Carcinoma of the inguinal nodes from a carcinoma of the vulva. The primary lesion was small. The presenting complaint was the ulcerated mass in the groin.

98 Vulval carcinoma. A carcinoma of the anterior part of the vulva and clitoral area. A metal catheter is in position to indicate how close the carcinoma is to the urethra. When the tumours are situated in this area, there is less chance of local recurrence if part of the urethra is excised during a radical vulvectomy operation.

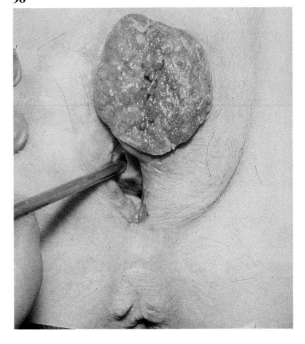

The urethra

The urethra is subject to infection by similar organisms to those which cause cystitis or pyelonephritis. In many instances, organisms which are present in the outer third of the urethra, without symptoms, produce symptoms when they are introduced into the bladder. The principle organisms which are of interest to the gynaecologist are, the gonococcus and the trichomonas. In any suspected case of gonorrhoea it is essential to take urethral swabs. Specific tests for syphilis should also be carried out before any broad spectrum antibiotics are given for suspected gonorrhoea.

Prolapse of the urethral mucosa most commonly occurs in the post-menopausal era, but can also occur in children. Although it can be acute, it is more often chronic. It is, in general, symptomless until it becomes traumatised or infected. If infected, it has to be distinguished from other causes of urethritis, caruncle, pseudocaruncle or carcinoma.

True caruncles are not all that common, and often the diagnosis is given incorrectly to a pseudocaruncle. The latter occurs as a result of a chronic urethritis, often due to chronic trichomoniasis infection. The true caruncle is an extremely vascular polyp attached to the posterior lip of the urethra. The tumour is, in essence, due to an eversion of the urethral mucosa. It has a varied histological picture depending on its constituents and the degree of infection which it usually presents. Clinically, it is tender to touch and scarlet in appearance.

The pseudocaruncle, or granulomatous caruncle, is a relatively localised form of chronic urethritis which affects not only the posterior lip of the urethra but extends around the sides as well. It is duller in appearance than a true caruncle and is not tender. In the majority of cases it represents a chronic trichomoniasis infection, but it can also be secondary to infection of prolapsed urethral mucosa.

Carcinoma of the urethra is uncommon as a primary lesion, but the urethra can often be secondarily involved in the extension of a vulval carcinoma. It is important for it to be diagnosed early, since its lymphatic spread is similar to the vulva. Most tumours are epithelial, arising from the transitional epithelium, rarely does one encounter an adenocarcinoma from the para-urethral glands.

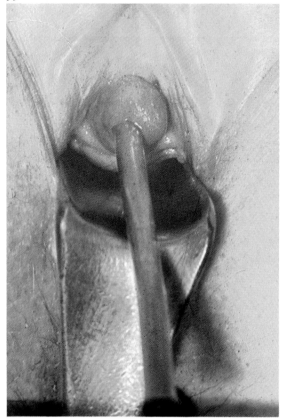

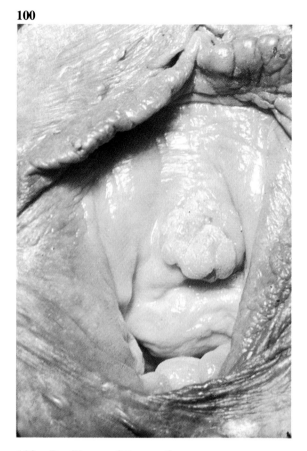

99 Prolapse of urethral mucosa. A catheter is in position. It can be treated by ligating the excess tissue and allowing it to slough off. It is, however, generally better to excise the excess tissue and to reconstitute the raw areas.

100 Papilloma of the urethra

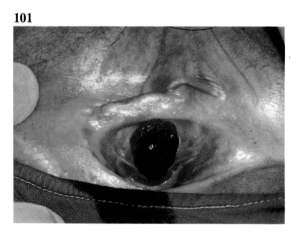

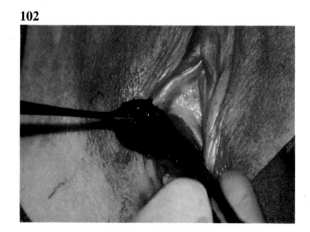

101 Urethral caruncle. This was extremely tender to touch. It was very vascular and the darker area had been traumatised and had bled.

102 Urethral caruncle. The caruncle shown in **101** being excised at its base. Histologically, there was a considerable amount of angiomatous tissue present.

103

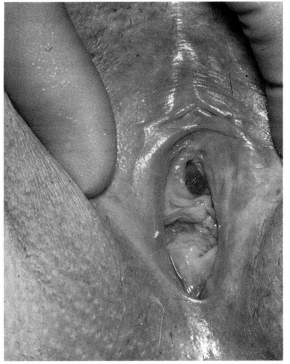

103 Urethral caruncle. This was very tender to touch and the principle complaint was dyspareunia. There had been no bleeding. Characteristically, they arise from the posterior lip of the urethra and have a narrow base.

105

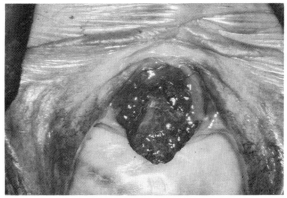

105 Prolapsed urethral mucosa: another example. It is associated with atrophic vaginitis.

104

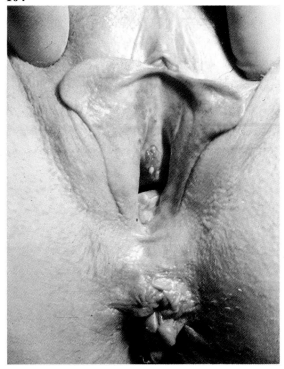

104 A pseudocaruncle associated with chronic trichomoniasis infection. It was not tender to touch.

106

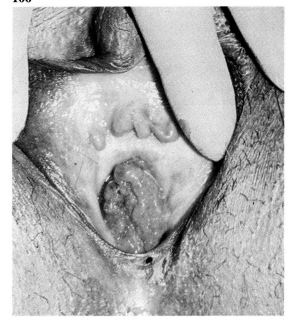

106 Carcinoma of the urethra. A polypoidal mass appearing at the urethra. The true diagnosis could easily be missed if not biopsied.

The vagina

From the gynaecological point of view, the vagina passes upwards and backwards from the vulva to the uterus, nearly parallel to the plane of the pelvic brim. Its anatomical relation to other structures in the pelvis, plus the fact that one can palpate pelvic contents through the fornices is perhaps more important to the gynaecologist than the pathological conditions which affect it.

The bladder and uterus are related to the anterior fornix, unless the uterus is retroverted. The lateral fornices are related to the fallopian tubes, ovaries, ureters, appendix and colon. The normal ovary, or slightly enlarged ovary, can be palpated in the lateral fornix, but large ovarian tumours, or cysts, move to the midline in the pelvis or abdomen. The fallopian tubes are never palpable, unless enlarged or thickened. The round ligament, which is of similar size, and runs in a similar direction, is sometimes mistaken for a fallopian tube.

An inflamed appendix may be difficult to distinguish in the right fornix from salpingitis, although the latter usually affects both tubes. Other gynaecological swellings in the lateral fornix include tubal pregnancy, broad ligament swellings, hydro – or pyosalpinges. On the right side, the caecum may be palable, and on the left, the pelvic or sigmoid colon. It is possible to palpate through the posterior fornix: the body of a retroverted uterus, with or without prolapsed ovaries, tumours of the uterus or ovary, blood or pus in the Pouch of Douglas, the uterosacral ligament and rectum.

The vagina does not have a secretion. The 'normal' discharge consists of exfoliated cells which accumulate in the vagina, and to which some cervical mucus, Doederlein bacilli and vaginal transudate are added to form a small amount of whitish acid material resembling curdled milk. This constitutes the normal discharge and should not be taken for pathological discharge.

The vagina is under hormonal influence during the reproductive era and the amount of normal discharge may vary slightly throughout the menstrual cycle, during hormone therapy and pregnancy. The vagina of a young girl before puberty and the older woman after the menopause is less resistant to infection than in the reproductive era, when the vagina is under oestrogen influence.

In relation to primary or secondary malignant tumours of the vagina, it is important to remember the development of the vagina. The upper two thirds of the vagina develop from the Mullerian ducts and the lymphatics from this area drain to the internal and external iliac lymph nodes, whereas the lower third, derived from the urogenital sinus, drains to the inguinal lymph nodes. The posterior vaginal wall lymphatics also drain into the nodes in the rectovaginal septum.

Some of the lesions or conditions in the following section might be considered vulval or cervical. The decision to include them has been arbitrary since many conditions involve, or spread to, the vagina when the primary condition originates from the vulva or cervix. For example, retained blood with a haematocolpos has already been illustrated in the section on the vulva, but it could have been included here.

Vaginitis often arises from vulval sources, or involves both the vagina and vulva as in vulvovaginitis. Malignant tumours in the vagina are more often secondary from the cervix, vulva or uterus, but can be from other sites. Prolapse and vaginal cysts are obviously included in this section. Apart from these conditions and tumours, the inclusion of the other conditions is perhaps debatable. They are, however, gynaecological and need to be included in this Atlas.

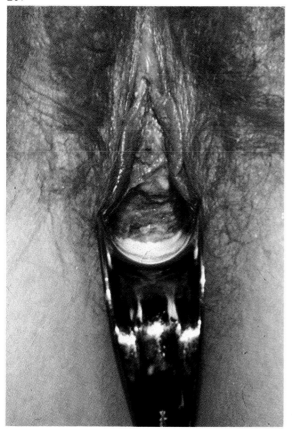

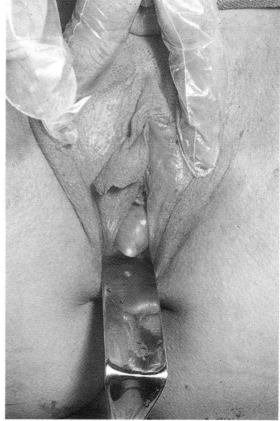

107 Monilial vaginitis with typical discharge, which is white and thick and often said to be similar to cream cheese in appearance. The more chronic infections have plaques of the discharge firmly attached to the vagina and if removed leave a raw area which bleeds.

108 An anterior vaginal wall cyst. It probably represents a residual remnant of the Wolffian duct. It is removed surgically and nowadays preferably marsupialised.

109

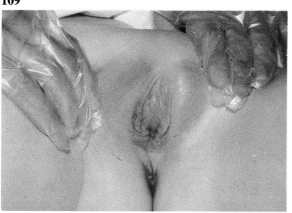

109 Testicular feminisation syndrome: The vaginal orifice and vulva of a 'woman' showing two lateral grooves on each side of the introitus which are not normally seen in the vulva. There is a small pigmented plaque at the lower end of the left labia minora which was histologically found to be a benign melanoma. The urogenital sinus in this patient was well developed, although the Mullerian duct system was, of course, absent.

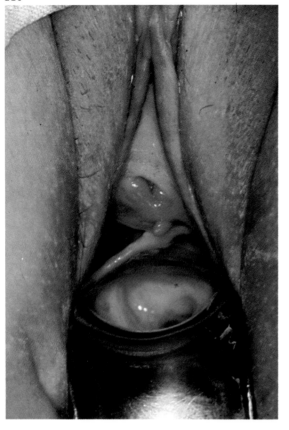

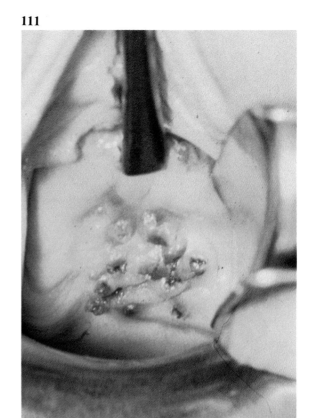

112

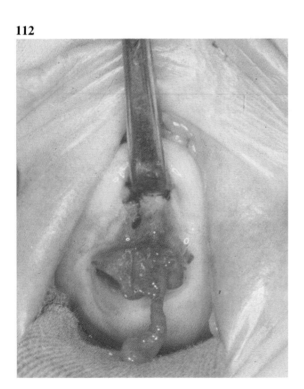

110 A vaginal septum. The speculum is inserted into the wider vagina. This patient had a well-developed Mullerian duct system on the left and a poorly developed one on the right. The septum had been missed previously when a bivalve speculum was used. Part of the left cervix can be visualised.

111 Endometriosis of the cervix. The ectopic areas of endometrial tissue are seen as blue areas on the posterior lip of the cervix. Some of these have broken down and are bleeding.

112 A first degree uterine prolapse. Even with traction, the cervix only just comes down to the introitus and not through it. The patient also has polyps protruding through the cervix. Histology revealed that both cervical and endometrial polyps were present. The treatment of this type of case is either a Manchester Repair or preferably a repair operation with vaginal hysterectomy. The patient has an adhesive plaster drape applied to the vulva.

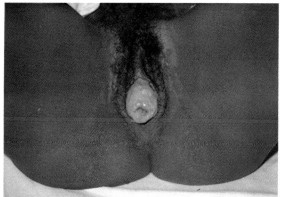

113 A second degree uterine prolapse. The cervix has passed through the introitus. The skin is dry and shows changes of keratinisation as a result of having been outside the vagina for sometime.

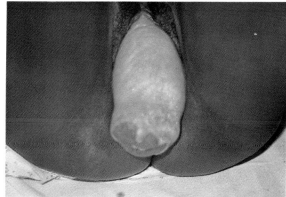

114 A third degree uterine prolapse or procidentia. The whole uterus and vaginal walls are outside the vagina. This occurred in a premenopausal patient of high parity.

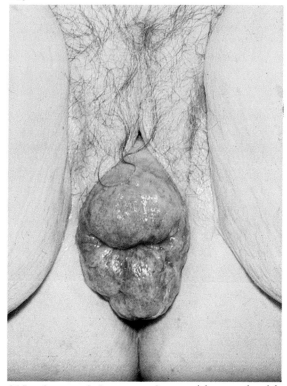

115 A second degree prolapse with an unhealthy cervix. This was traumatised as a result of being outside the vagina and the patient complained of bleeding as well as 'something coming down'. Cervical cytology was abnormal and histologically dysplasia was present. There was no evidence of malignancy.

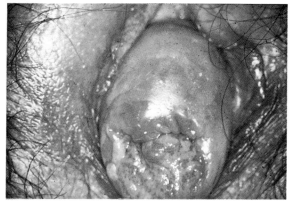

116 A second degree prolapse. A closer view of the cervix in a patient with prolapse. It is easy to appreciate that bleeding is likely to occur if the epithelium of this cervix is traumatised.

117

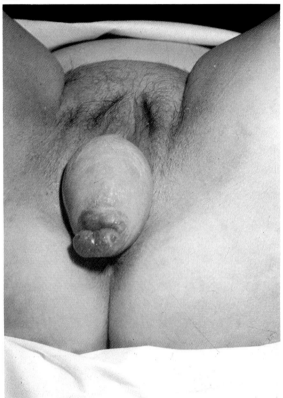

118

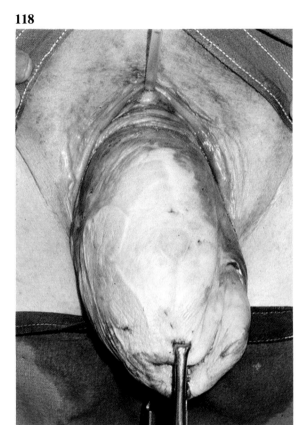

117 A procidentia. The anterior wall with the bladder behind is easy to visualise. The anterior lip of the cervix shows evidence of keratinisation compared to the posterior lip.

118 A procidentia which reveals marked keratinisation of the vaginal skin, compared with the upper portions which have remained inside the introitus. This is revealed as a result of traction on the cervix.

119

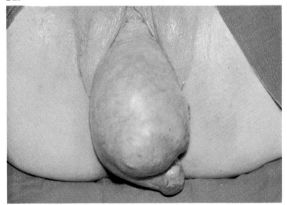

120

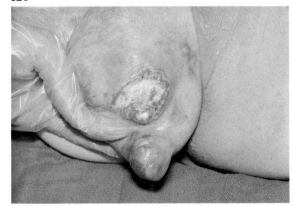

119 Vault prolapse with slight ulceration on the left side. Although it looks as if the cervix is present, it is not. The patient had an abdominal total hysterectomy 15 years previously. There were small loops of bowel present in this prolapse.

120 Vault prolapse in **119** rotated to reveal the ulcerated area. The part which looks like the cervix is the inverted vault of the vagina. It probably represents the weakest part of the vaginal vault following the previous abdominal hysterectomy.

121 Ectopia vesica repair and prolapse. The ectopia was repaired when the patient was a child. The prolapse developed later in life.

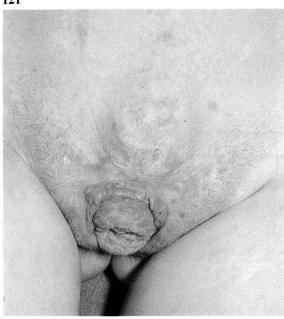

122 Ectopia vesica repair and prolapse. The prolapse is more apparent and the separated labia can be seen. There is a small polyp in the cervical canal. This is the same patient as in **121**, but in this instance, the patient was straining. There is also herniation of the abdominal incision.

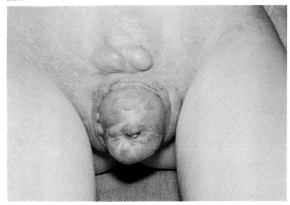

123 Uterovaginal prolapse and rectal prolapse. The rectal prolapse is more marked than the second degree uterine prolapse. An elderly patient who responded well to surgery of both conditions.

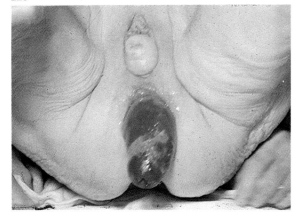

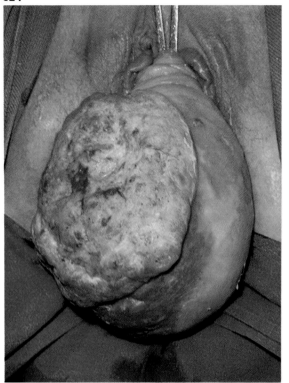

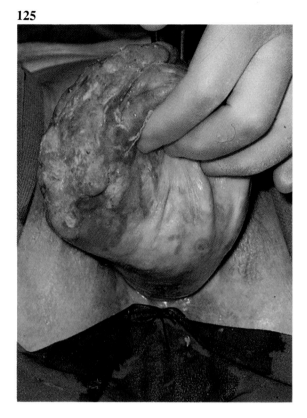

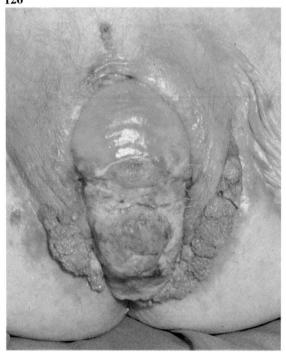

124   A procidentia with a large epithelioma. Behind the carcinoma is the bladder. The patient had been too embarrassed to attend until she was no longer capable of looking after herself.

125   Carcinoma of the vagina plus a procidentia. The prolapse shown in **124** has been elevated. Instead of bowel being present behind the small uterus as would be expected, there was bladder! There had obviously been incomplete emptying of the bladder. In essence, part of the bladder was in the normal position anterior to the uterus, but the major part had passed over the fundus of the uterus to occupy the Pouch of Douglas. As a result of the stasis there was a urinary infection present.

126   Vaginal   carcinoma,   procidentia   and condylomata. The necrotic neoplastic process on the vagina is typical of an epithelioma of squamous cell origin. The vulval masses were not secondary involvement   but   histologically   condylomata contrary to the clinical impression of secondary tumour.

127 Vaginal prolapse plus carcinoma of the vulva. This woman was 90 years of age and looked after herself in all respects. Vaginal hysterectomy and wide resection relieved all her symptoms, and she resumed her normal activities. She was alive and well two years later without evidence of recurrence.

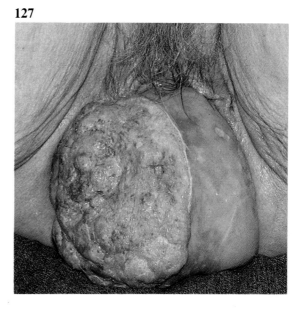

128 Vaginal atresia. This patient has only the lower part of the vagina developed with an absent uterus. A catheter has been inserted prior to a William's vaginoplasty operation.

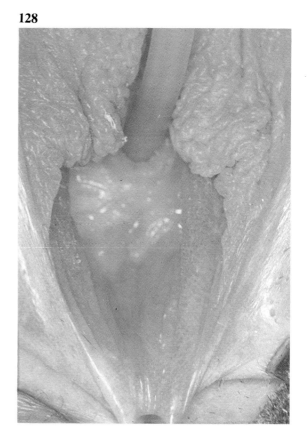

129

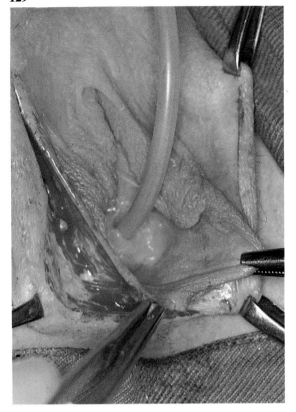

130

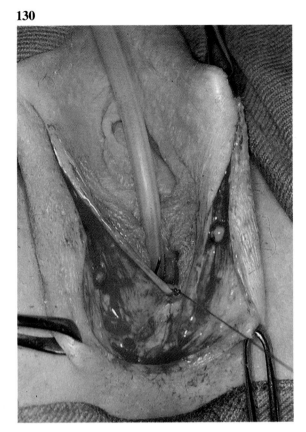

131

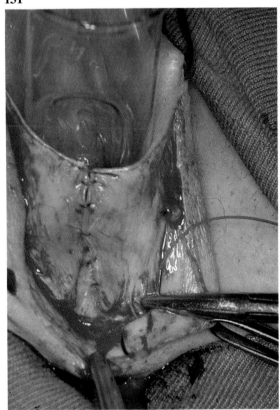

129 Vaginoplasty. The first stage in the formation of an artificial vagina. The incision is made outside the labia minora.

130 Vaginoplasty. The second stage involves suturing the inner skin incisions.

131 Vaginoplasty. The vaginal dilator has been inserted into the artificial vaginal pouch and the muscles are being approximated.

132

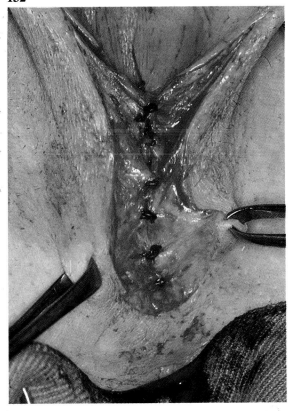

133

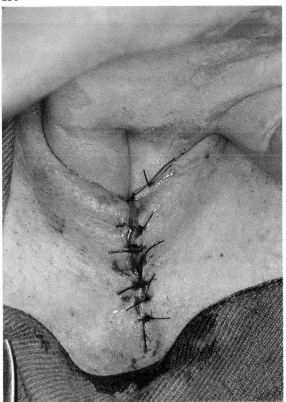

134

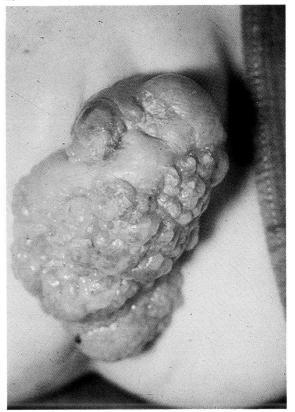

132   Vaginoplasty. The muscles and deeper tissues have been approximated.

133   Vaginoplasty. The completed operation shows the width and length of the vagina on vaginal examination.

134   Sarcoma botryoides. This tumour in a young girl originated in the vagina and protruded through the introitus. It is uncommon. The tumour is usually more haemorrhagic than appears in this case.

135 Clear cell adenocarcinoma. *(Colposcopy × 16).* A very haemorrhagic tumour. The principle symptoms were intermenstrual bleeding and post-coital bleeding. There was a history of DES exposure in utero.

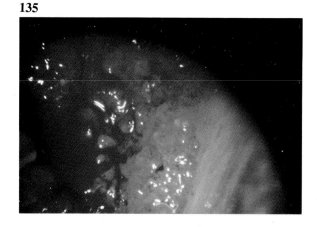

136 Clear cell carcinoma of the vagina. *(Colposcopy × 25).* The same case as **135** at a higher magnification. These photographs are taken five weeks after progestogen therapy. The original appearance of the tumour is shown in **390**.

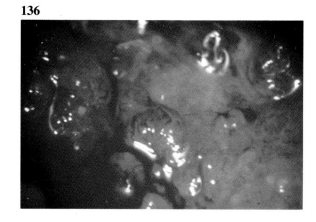

137 Clear cell adenocarcinoma of the vagina. The post-operative specimen which shows the packed vagina closed off, uterus and appendages. The pelvic wall nodes and parametrial tissue were removed separately and are not shown in this specimen.

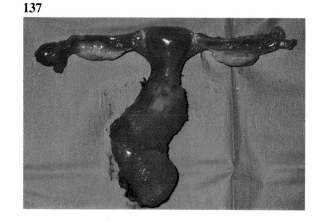

The cervix

Cervicitis strictly refers to infection of the cervical glands, the deeper tissue of the cervix and the endocervix. Infections of the cervix can occur as part of a vaginitis, but are excluded from the term cervicitis. Whilst cervicitis may be acute or chronic, the latter is more common. Acute cervicitis occurs as a consequence of surgical or obstetrical trauma. Puerperal or gonococcal infections also produce acute cervicitis, but the infections and symptoms in other parts of the genital tract always cause more concern.

Syphilitic infection and sexually transmitted diseases, other than gonorrhoea, may affect the cervix. Tuberculosis of the genital tract can also involve the cervix.

Chronic cervicitis is common as a histological finding. Many symptoms which are said to be related to chronic cervicitis are really related to infection of the adjacent parametrial tissues. The only symptom which can be specifically related to chronic cervicitis is discharge.

The length of the cervix is variable, but it may appear elongated in comparison to a short vagina. The commonest cause of elongation of the supra-vaginal portion of the cervix is uterine prolapse.

Benign tumours or cysts may arise in the cervix, whilst malignant tumours may be primary or secondary. Conditions which arise in the uterus may spread to the cervix or pass through the cervical canal. Many of these are considered in this section since they are visible.

The epithelium of the cervix is under hormonal influence during the reproductive era of a woman's life and undergoes cyclical changes. There is a junctional zone at the external os where the columnar epithelium of the cervical canal changes over to squamous epithelium. The precise site of change is variable, but it is vulnerable to physical and chemical changes. The cervix is liable to trauma from a variety of causes, including coitus, childbearing and gynaecological procedures. Since the cervix is available for inspection, many of the changes can be noted and are therefore included in this section.

The hope that cervical carcinoma can be reduced by cervical cytology has not generally been realised. In certain areas and countries, however, the diagnosis has been made at an earlier stage. Early carcinomas shown in this section have not been grouped together deliberately, in order that the reader will be aware how easy it is for the diagnosis to be missed. Early diagnosis of carcinoma is of considerable benefit to the patient and her family. One should always remember that the symptoms of carcinoma of the cervix are late. The process starts in the basal layers of the epidermis. Micro-invasion occurs by penetration through the basal layers of the epidermis and somewhat later the superficial layers of the epidermis are broken. Only then will symptoms such as contact bleeding or discharge occur. When these symptoms do occur, the lesion is already Stage I or II.

138

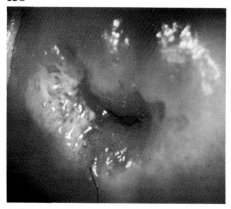

138 Early carcinoma of the cervix. A small central erosion with a whitish area between 7 and 10 o'clock. Not obviously malignant to the naked eye, but should be considered suspicious. Cervical smear revealed malignant cells.

139

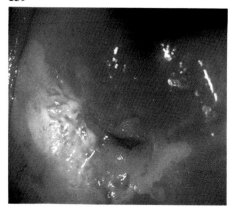

139 Schiller's iodine applied to the cervix in 138. The whitish area does not stain: the test is positive. A few puntate red areas are noticed which are typical of neoplasia. Biopsy confirmed invasive carcinoma of the cervix clinically Stage I.

140

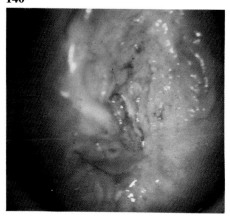

140 Carcinoma of the cervix. Characteristic appearance of an early carcinoma of the cervix. Diagnosed on routine examination in pregnancy. The patient had noticed some increase in discharge but thought it was 'normal'. It is doubtful if she would have attended if she was not pregnant.

141 Polypoidal proliferation noted in the last month of pregnancy. Appearances suggest a polyp.

142 The appearances of the cervix shown in **141** three months later at the postnatal clinic. No evidence of the polypoidal tissue.

141

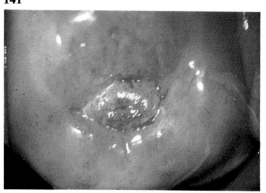

142

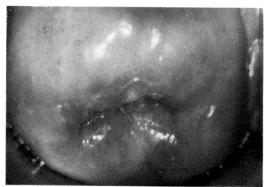

143 Cervical polyp found in pregnancy. The patient had a small blood loss (postcoital) at six months gestation. No other cause of bleeding was found.

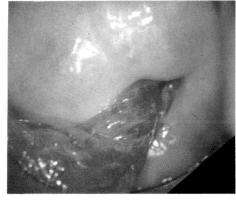

144 Cervical polyps noted in early pregnancy. Symptomless, found on routine speculum examination.

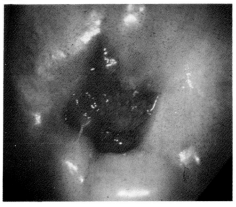

145 Postnatal examination of the same cervix (144). No evidence of polyp, healthy cervix.

146 Lacerated cervix noted in early pregnancy at eight weeks. Normal cervical smear.

147 Lacerated cervix. The same cervix (146) at thirty-two weeks gestation. A marked change in the appearances reflecting the hormonal changes.

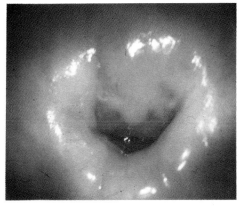

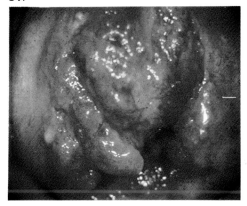

148

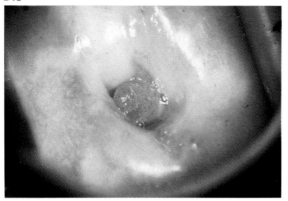

148 Cervical polyp found in early pregnancy. It was symptomless.

149

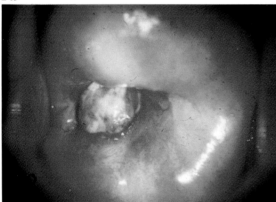

149 Infected cervical polyp. A mucopurulent discharge is seen over the polyp protruding through the cervical canal.

150

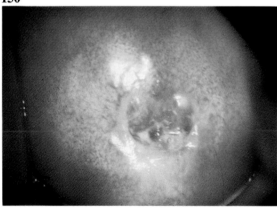

150 Monilial infection of the cervix. The cervix is covered in the central area with whitened plaque of discharge associated with a monilial infection. An occluded cervical gland is visible at 1 o'clock near the cervical os.

151 Bleeding cervical erosion found at eight weeks gestation. Small amount of blood seen in the region of the canal and superficially near the edge of the speculum.

152 Cervical erosion. Appearances following electrocautery.

151

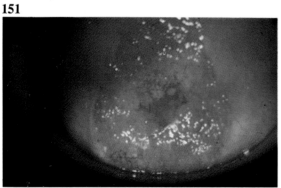

152

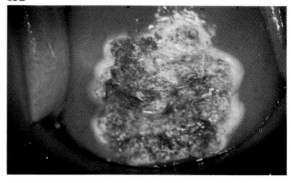

153 Cervical erosion – appearance of the cervix in **152**, twelve weeks after electrocautery to the cervix. Normal appearances.

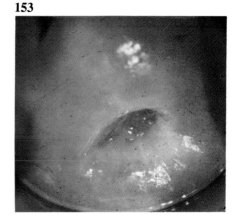

154 Punch biopsies of the cervix. The appearances after punch biopsies on the anterior and posterior lips of the cervix.

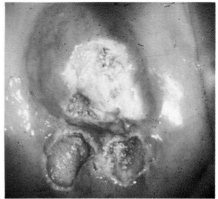

155 Punch biopsies of the cervix. Appearances of the cervix in **154** are normal when seen twelve weeks later.

156 Chorionepithelioma of the cervix. A secondary deposit on the cervix. A haemorrhagic tumour with a few darker areas.

157 Punch biopsies of the cervix. Biopsy of the cervix taken from a woman with condylomata of the vulva and cervix in early pregnancy. The main lesions only were biopsied to confirm the diagnosis.

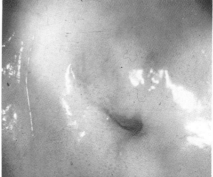

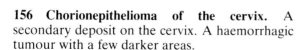

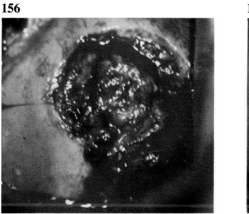

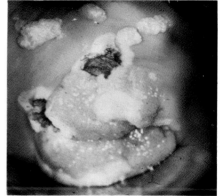

158

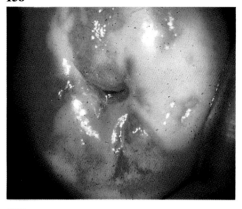

158 Staphylococcal infection of the cervix secondary to the vagina. There are some raw areas and some healing areas. There was no evidence of a superadded monilial infection despite the white areas on the cervix.

159

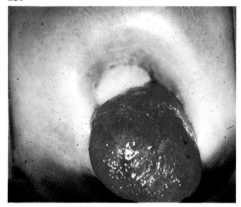

159 Cervical polyp. A small plug of cotton wool has been placed on the external os to display the polyp.

160

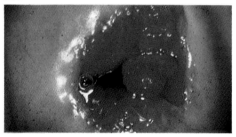

160 Lacerated cervix with erosion and polypoidal projection. It is impossible to tell from the picture whether there is a discrete polyp. In fact, there was, and it arose from higher in the cervical canal.

161

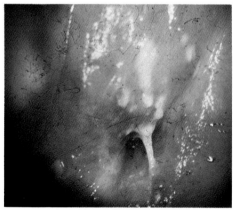

161 An infected cervix with mucopurulent discharge present on the cervix and over the external os.

162   A cervix six weeks after diathermy. Although not completely healed the cervical canal appears more like that of a nulliparous patient.

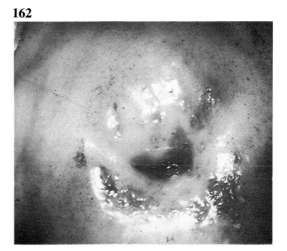

163   A lacerated and eroded cervix.

163

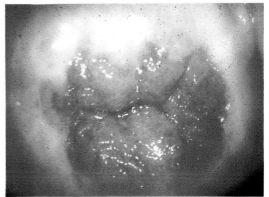

164   Atresia of the cervical os. This was noted in a postmenopausal woman who had atrophic changes in the vulval area. There is a small dimple where the cervical os had probably been situated.

164

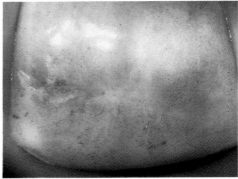

165   Atresia of the cervical os following the menopause. It is sometimes associated with pyometra as in this case.

166   Atrophic vaginitis and cervical polyps. The cervix had undergone atrophic changes, but it is not easy to see. The cervix was very short and nearly flush with the vaginal vault.

165

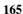
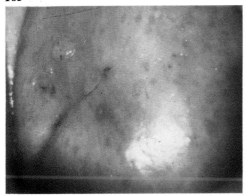

166

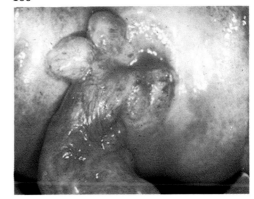

167

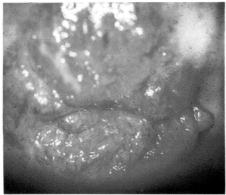

167 Cervical erosion and polypoidal proliferation. The latter appears to be almost cystic at about 3 o'clock. This is in contrast to the appearance at about 9 o'clock.

168

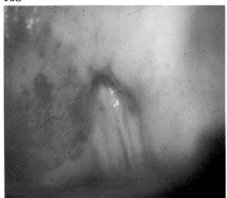

168 Early carcinoma of the cervix. Despite the difference in appearance this is the same cervix as **167** but five years later. Extensive diathermy had been applied shortly after the picture shown in **167** had been taken. The area at 9 o'clock bled on touching and a small amount of blood can be seen in the mucoid discharge coming from the cervical canal.

169

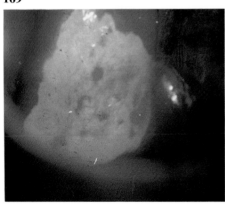

169 Schiller's iodine applied to the cervix from 168. The area on the right of the cervical os fails to stain with iodine.

170 Early carcinoma of the cervix. Biopsy of **168**. The diagnosis was confirmed histologically as a squamous cell carcinoma and clinically a Stage I carcinoma.

171 Chronic cervicitis. A large number of Nabothian follicles are present. The cervical glands and ducts have become occluded forming the characteristic 'blue-domed cysts'.

170

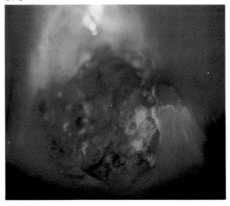

171

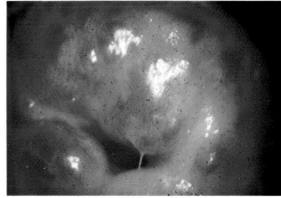

172 Erosion of the cervix. This was taken at the time of ovulation. An impression is given of the clear cervical mucus. There is a small bubble on the left side.

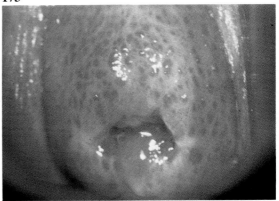

173 Trichomoniasis of the cervix. The typical appearance can be made out. There is also some clear mucus coming out of the cervical canal.

174 Treated trichomoniasis of the vagina and cervix. Following effective treatment there should be complete resolution of the lesions. This picture was taken immediately after the completion of treatment in order to show the change from **173**.

175 A glycogen free area of the anterior lip of the cervix.

176 Biopsy from glycogen free area from patient in **175** but showing the stain after the biopsy had been taken. There was no evidence of malignancy, metaplasia only was found in the specimen.

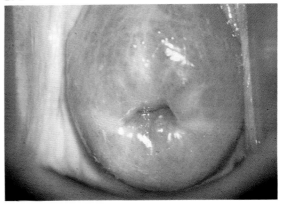

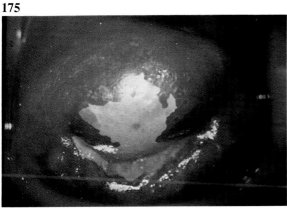

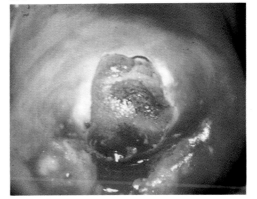

177

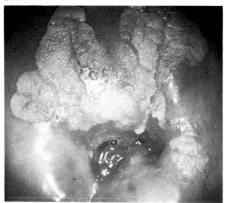

177 Leucoplakia of the cervix. There were similar appearances on the vulva and vagina. There was no evidence of malignancy in the biopsies taken.

178

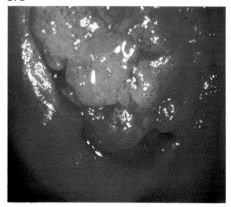

178 Carcinoma of the cervix. There is some bleeding from the lesion. The irregularity is quite marked and there is loss of normal contours and appearances.

179

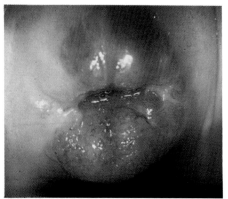

179 Laceration of the cervix. The posterior lip reveals the patterns often seen within the cervical canal. The only symptom was of vaginal discharge.

180 Laceration of the cervix. A more marked laceration than shown on **179**. Sometimes referred to as **ectropion of the cervix**, which means the eversion of the cervical os with exposure of the cervical canal. A more definite arbor vitae pattern can be seen in the anterior and posterior lips. The principal symptom was vaginal discharge.

181 The cervical laceration shown in **180** was treated by cervical conisation. These appearances two years later show a marked improvement. The patient had no vaginal discharge.

180

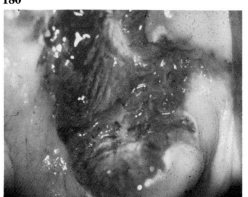

181

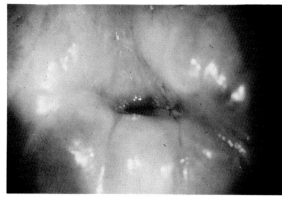

182   Lacerated cervix shown to indicate the variation. The whole cervix was firm in consistency. If an attempt is made to put a sound into the lacerated area it would meet resistance. If inserted into a carcinoma, the sound would penetrate the tumour rather like a ripe pear.

182

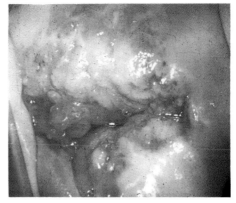

183   Solitary Nabothian follicle on posterior lip. There is a smaller but similar swelling inside the canal on the inner aspect of the anterior lip of the cervix.

183

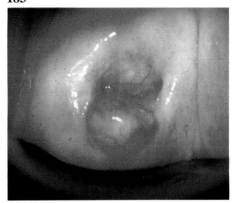

184   Chancre of cervix. Unusual to see nowadays, but has to be considered. Punched out ulcer on anterior lip at approximately 12 o'clock and another between 10 and 11 o'clock.

185   Cervical infection. This patient had a cervical erosion with superadded infection. As a result, the erosion bled on contact.

186   Treated cervical infection with local antibiotic cream. The cervix shown in **185** ten weeks after treatment. The large area noted previously has regressed and has healed. There is a small central erosion.

184

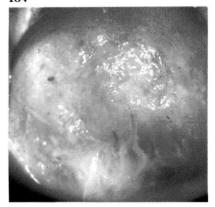

185

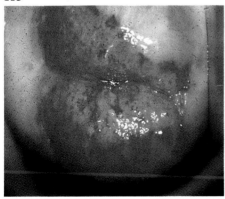

186

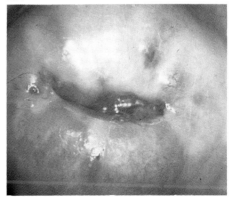

187

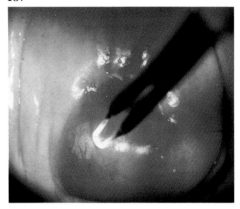

187   Electrocautery about to be applied to a large Nabothian follicle on the posterior lip of the cervix.

188

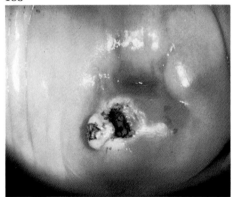

188   Cautery of Nabothian follicle. The material present is at the site of the cauterised follicle.

189

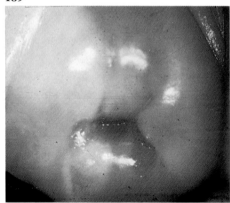

189   Cautery of Nabothian follicle. The appearance of **187** two months later. It is now healed, although the site of the cautery can still be identified.

190   Radical electrocautery of the cervix. The immediate effects of the cautery incisions can be made out.

191   Multiple radical cautery: appearance of **190** four months later. The cervix looks normal and there is no evidence of previous cautery.

190

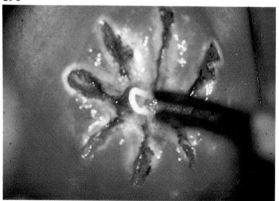

191

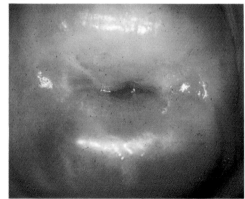

192   Leucoplakia of the cervix. A central erosion surrounded by a white area which is more marked on the anterior lip.

192

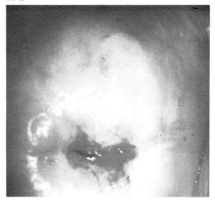

193   Schiller's iodine applied to areas of leukoplakia of the cervix shown in **192**. The areas are glycogen free. There are no abnormal vascularities.

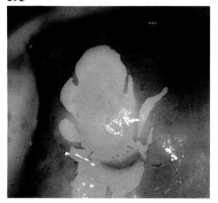

194   Chronic cervicitis. A large amount of mucopurulent discharge can be seen coming out of the cervical canal.

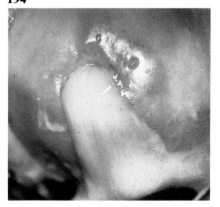

195   An early invasive carcinoma of the posterior lip of the cervix. Small amounts of blood can be seen on the area of abnormality.

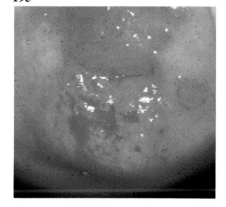

196

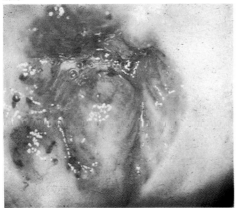

196 **A lacerated cervix** with secretions visible from the exposed cervical mucosa.

197

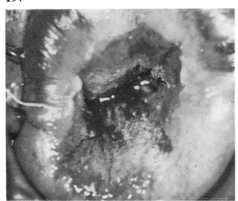

197 **The immediate appearance of conisation** of the lacerated cervix in **196**.

198

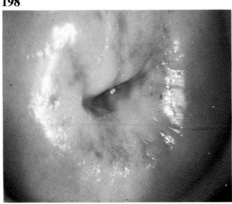

198 **The cervix from 196** nine months later after conisation without suturing the area.

199 **Cervical erosion and polyps.** The polyp is central but the polypoidal mass on the right is related to the erosion.

200 **An early invasive carcinoma.** Again the area with blood should arouse suspicion. The cervical smear revealed malignant cells and the diagnosis was confirmed by biopsy.

200

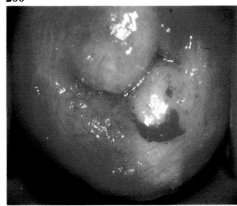

199

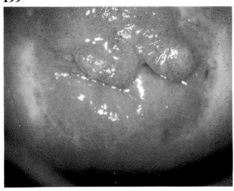

201 Early invasive carcinoma. The cervix, despite appearing virtually normal, has an early carcinoma present at the external os. A cervical smear revealed malignant cells and biopsy confirmed the diagnosis. Lesions were present on both anterior and posterior lips of the cervix.

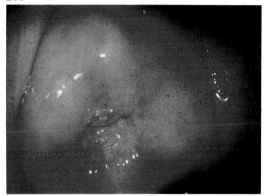

202 Leucoplakia of the cervix. The patient had no symptoms. Leucoplakia was noted when a cervical smear was taken, although the smear itself revealed no abnormality.

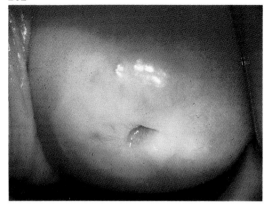

203 Schiller's iodine applied to leucoplakia of the cervix shown in **202**. Part of the leucoplakic area takes up iodine and part does not.

204 Biopsy site from glycogen free area. The biopsy revealed no evidence of any malignancy.

205 The healed biopsy area from the cervix shown in **202**, **203** and **204**. The leucoplakia being less apparent than when first seen in **202**.

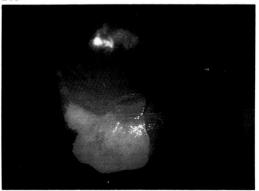

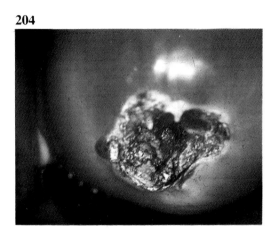

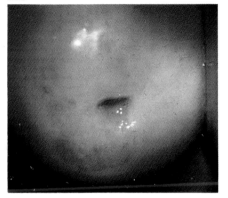

206

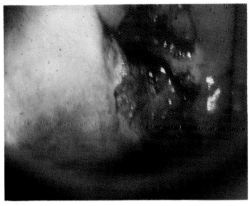

206   A carcinoma of the cervix. An ulcerated area with obvious blood. The diagnosis was easily made on clinical grounds.

207

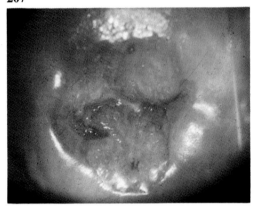

207   Carcinoma *in situ* of the cervix. An ulcerated cervix noted in pregnancy, which was suggestive of carcinoma but histology only revealed carcinoma *in situ*. Smears revealed malignant cells. A cone biopsy was carried out without any complications. The patient had an otherwise uneventful pregnancy and labour ended in a spontaneous vaginal delivery.

208

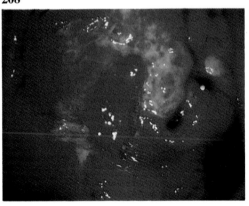

208   Tuberculosis of the cervix. This might be mistaken for a carcinoma but does not usually have the friability of a carcinoma. The diagnosis was confirmed histologically and by culture.

209

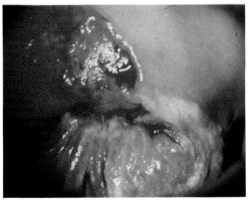

209   Carcinoma of the cervix. A small portion shows leucoplakic appearances on the left. This was clinically diagnosed as a Stage II cervical carcinoma and was treated by radiotherapy.

210 Granuloma inguinale. The unusual appearance of the cervix probably represents the beginning of healing by fibrosis, which is characteristic of this disease. Fibrosis and distortion of the tissue involved is a feature. More often involves the vulva.

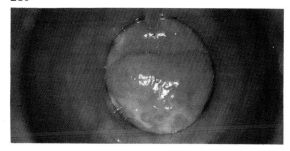

211 Granuloma inguinale of the cervix: a closer view of **210**. There is some distortion of the normal tissues.

211

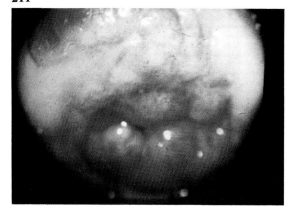

212 Tuberculosis of the cervix. Two discrete lesions are visible. The patient was a known case of tuberculosis and was treated before effective therapy was available 20 years prior to this diagnosis being made. Principle symptoms: vaginal discharge and infertility. The latter was due to tuberculous salpingitis which was also present.

213 Endometriosis of the cervix. The dark area at 3 o'clock had been noted to increase in size in the pre-menstrual phase of the menstrual cycle.

214 Early carcinoma of the cervix. The lesion just above the external os extends on the cervix, but no further. It was clinically staged as I and treated surgically by a Wertheim's hysterectomy operation. There was no involvement of the pelvic wall nodes.

212

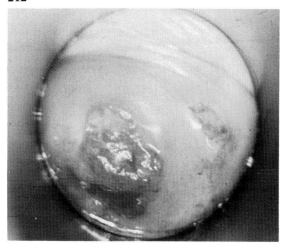

213

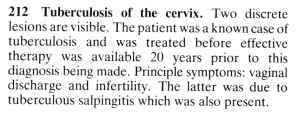

214

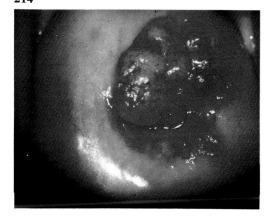

215

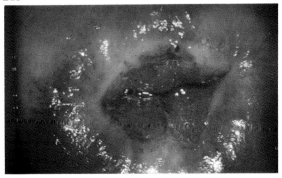

215 An early carcinoma of the cervix. The appearance is somewhat deceptive and reveals the importance of carrying out cytology, colposcopy if available, and biopsy before excluding the diagnosis.

216

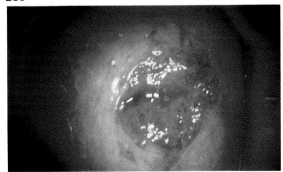

216 Microinvasion of the cervix. Clinically there was no suggestion of malignancy. Positive cytology. Colposcopy was, however, suggestive of carcinoma. A cone biopsy confirmed microinvasion and nowadays classified as Stage I.

217

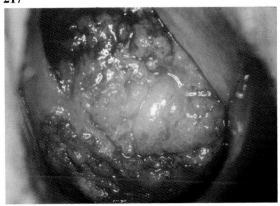

217 Carcinoma of the cervix. Clinically a Stage II carcinoma. The lesion is more typical in appearance and not likely to be missed.

218

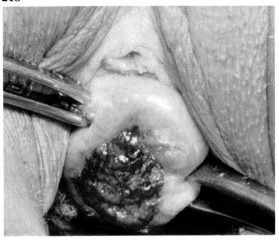

218 Tuberculosis of the cervix. The polypoidal mass could, perhaps, be mistaken for a carcinoma, but it was not friable. The diagnosis was confirmed histologically and by guinea pig inoculation.

219 Cervical polyp in labour. The polyp can be seen below the fetal head at full dilatation of the cervix.

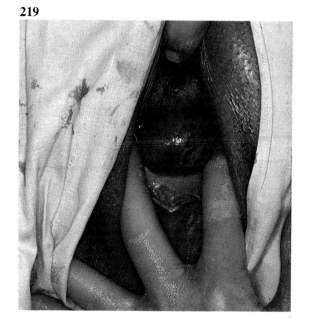

220 Trichomonas vaginalis infection. The typical discharge can be seen at the cervical os and in the posterior fornix. The greenish colour and the small bubbles are characteristic.

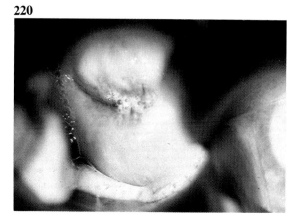

221 Pill ectopy. As a result of taking combined oestrogen and progestogen pills the columnar epithelium has replaced or overgrown the squamous epithelium. The effect in this case is more marked than usual.

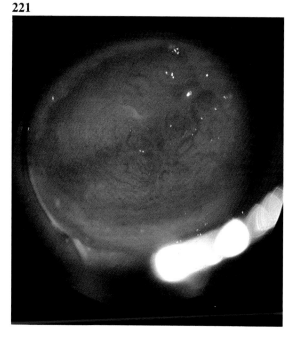

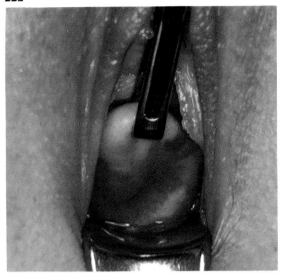

222 Carcinoma *in situ*. There is nothing visible other than a marked erosion of the cervix. Repeated abnormal cytology was followed by a cone biopsy. The absolute diagnosis can only be made on histological grounds.

223

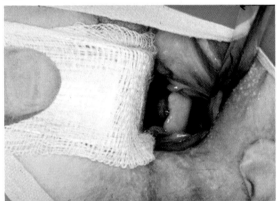

223 Congenital abnormality of the genital tract. The two vagina are exposed. The patient had a double genital tract throughout. The principle symptom of dysmenorrhoea was relieved by suppression of ovulation.

224

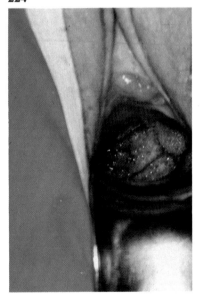

224 The cervix on the right side of the patient shown in **223**. The septum can be seen in view at the left side of this vagina.

225

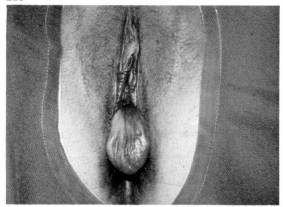

225 Cervical polyp. The polyp at the introitus is similar to a tongue in appearance.

226 Cervical polyp. The unusual length of the polyp shown in **225** was revealed when pulled out. The only complaint by the patient was of something coming down on standing or straining.

227 Cervical polyp. A large polyp which protrudes through the introitus and covers the anus.

228 Fibroid polyp protruding through the cervix. A bi-lobed pedunculated fibroid. The patient complained of heavy periods and sudden severe dysmenorrhoea. The latter presumably being due to the fibroid passing through the cervical canal.

229 Carcinoma of the cervix. An obvious carcinoma of the anterior lip of the cervix, which extended on to the vagina on the right side.

228

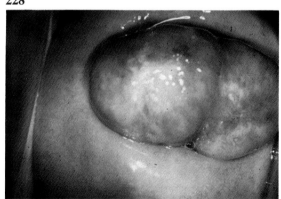

226

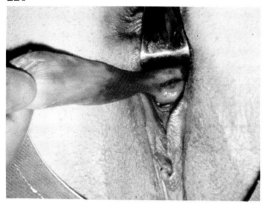

227

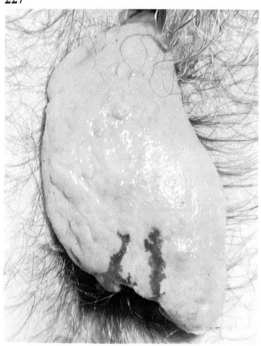

229

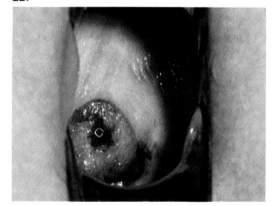

The uterus and appendages

As mentioned earlier, lesions of these structures cannot easily be visualised, and therefore are not considered in as much detail as conditions which can be visualised. The pelvic organs can be visualised at laparotomy, laparoscopy or culdoscopy and a few examples have been chosen.

Most gynaecological conditions of the uterus, fallopian tubes and ovaries, which are dealt with surgically, if of interest, are mounted in specimen pots and put into gynaecological museums. A study of these pots and their case histories is another useful method of obtaining knowledge of gynaecological pathology and gynaecology.

Lesions of the uterus and ovary which affect the size or position of these structures are diagnosed by abdominal and bimanual palpation. This skill cannot be learnt in books, even those containing pictures. Knowledge of the macroscopic changes is gained only by experience in the operating theatre and by the study of museum specimens, as well as from clinical practice.

With regard to the uterus, it is important to be able to determine its size, shape, consistency, position and mobility. The same applies to the ovaries, but it is also necessary to determine whether there are changes on one or both sides.

230 Submucous fibroid shown in a hysterectomy specimen. The colour of the submucous fibroid reflects the interference with its blood supply. It would also, from its size, have protruded through the cervix. This uterus is normal in size and the submucous polyp was seen protruding through the cervix on speculum examination and felt on bimanual examination.

230

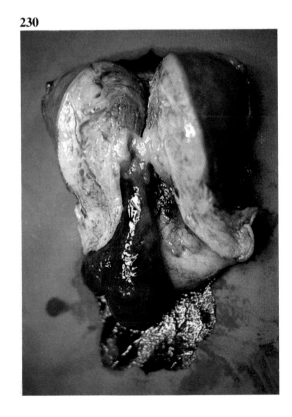

231

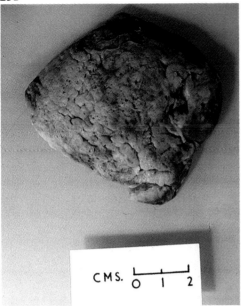

CMS. 0 1 2

231 A decidual cast. This was extruded from the uterus in a case of missed abortion. The patient had infrequent menstrual cycles and was not aware that she was pregnant. Her presenting symptom was sudden pain and she passed this cast and brought it in with her.

232

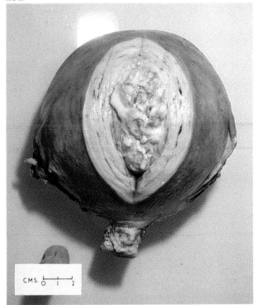

CMS. 0 1 2

232 Fibroid uterus. A uterus enlarged by a single fibroid. This patient complained of menorrhagia and dysmenorrhoea. The clinical diagnosis was adenomyosis or fibroids, but the symmetrical enlargement was considered to favour the former diagnosis.

233

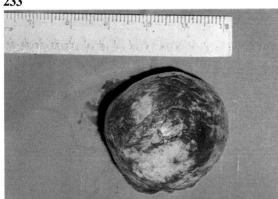

233 Uterine fibroid. The more typical appearance of a fibroid. This patient had a large single fibroid. Her only symptom was infertility. The specimen was obtained at a myomectomy operation. The patient subsequently had two pregnancies.

234 Stromal endometriosis. An unusual condition diagnosed histologically. This patient had menorrhagia and dysmenorrhoea. The reason for the enlarged uterus on clinical examination and history was considered to be adenomyosis. Some consider the condition to be a peculiar neoplastic variant of adenomyosis. Another view is that undifferentiated cells have the potential, when stimulated, to develop into either adenomyosis or stromal endometriosis.

234

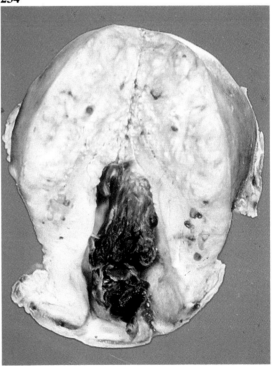

235 Cervical pregnancy. The specimen consists of an enlarged uterus with obvious placental tissues in the cervical canal and adherent on the right side. This is a rare form of ectopic gestation, and bleeding from the site is often severe enough, as in this case, for a hysterectomy to be performed. Although the quality of the picture is not good, it was decided to include it as it is an unusual condition.

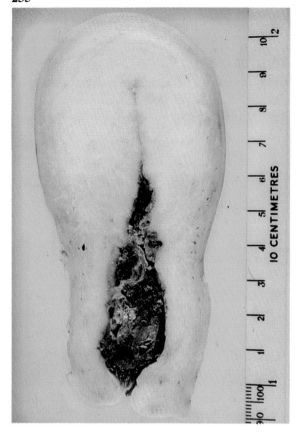

236 Carcinoma of the body of the uterus. The necrotic mass of tissue in the fundus of the uterus is easily made out. This patient had the typical symptom, namely, post-menopausal bleeding. The diagnosis was made by curettage when obvious malignant tissue was obtained. Normal healthy endometrium comes out in strips. Both appendages were removed and post-operative radiotherapy was given to the vagina.

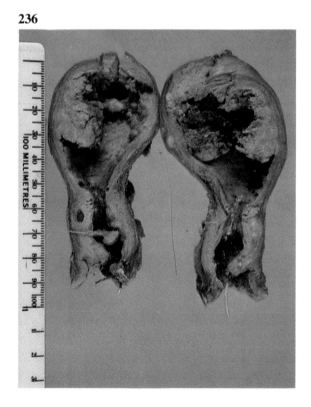

237 Carcinoma of the uterus. A small tumour in the fundus of the uterus with another nodule of tumour in the mid-line of the uterus. There was also secondary spread to the ovary on the left side.

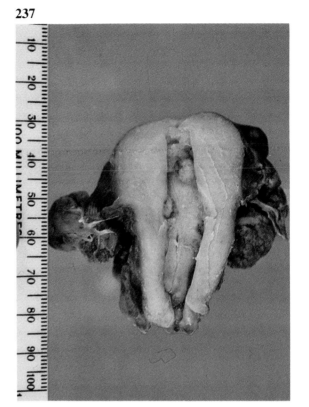

238 Bicornuate uterus. The appearances following delivery by Caesarean section. The right horn being most marked. The veins on both sides were more marked than usual. The ovaries are normal. This patient had no gynaecological symptoms and no difficulty in conceiving.

239 Bicornuate uterus with a common cervix, also called a uterus bicornis unicollis. There appears to be a polyp present, but this is not the case. It is the posterior lip of the cervix.

240 The uterus bicornis unicollis from 239 shown in a hysterogram.

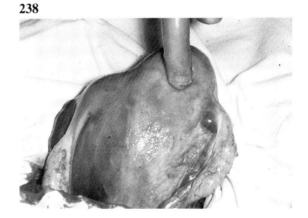

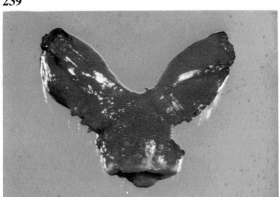

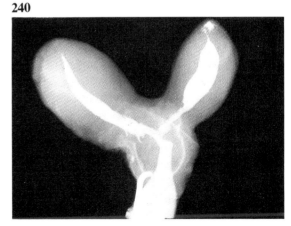

241

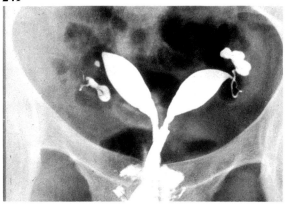

241   Uterus bicornis unicollis. Hysterosalpingogram showing the uterine cavities with dye in the fallopian tubes. There is also a leak of dye into the vagina. No free spill of dye in this particular salpingogram.

242

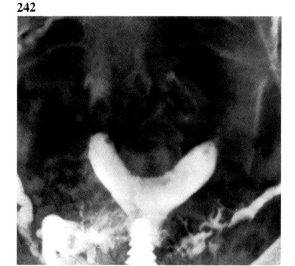

242   Bicornuate uterus. With this type of hysterogram it is important to remember that a similar picture would be obtained if there was a fibroid in the fundus. There is no apparent spill of dye in this picture, but the fallopian tubes were open and the patient conceived. The patient went into premature labour (had a live child) and retained placenta. Both recognised complications of uterine abnormalities. There is also some extravasation of dye into the blood vessels.

243

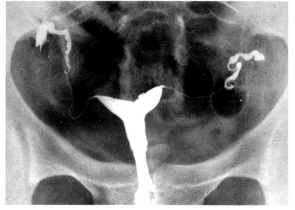

243   Uterine fibroid: Hysterosalpingogram reveals some irregularity in the fundal region. This uterus contained a fibroid in the fundal region and hence the defect in the uterine shape. There is free spill of dye on both sides.

244

244   The normal appearances of fallopian tubes in a hysterosalpingogram. There is a slight dip at the middle of the fundus, perhaps representing the site of fusion of the Mullerian ducts, or a mild bicornuate tendency. The inner parts of the fallopian tubes are narrow compared with the wider ampullary end.

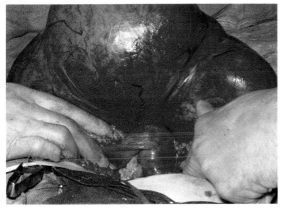

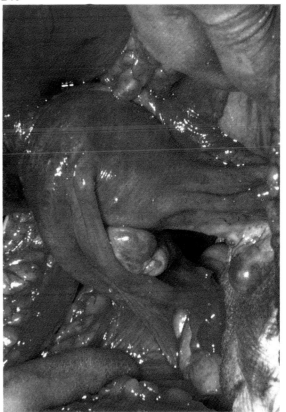

245   A broad ligament fibroid. The large mass corresponding to an 18 week pregnancy felt soft. There was considerable doubt about the diagnosis. Laparotomy revealed the uterus and left appendage to be rotated by the fibroid.

246   The broad ligament fibroid shown in **245** has been freed from its surroundings but not from the uterus. The fibroid is at the top left of the picture, attached to the uterus by a broad pedicle. Although the fibroid arose from the left side of the uterus, it had passed in front of the uterus under the uterovesical pouch of peritoneum into the broad ligament on the right. The operator's fingers indicates the position in which the fibroid was situated. It is perhaps not surprising that there was doubt about the diagnosis prior to laparotomy. The fibroid was covered by peritoneum throughout its course from one broad ligament to another.

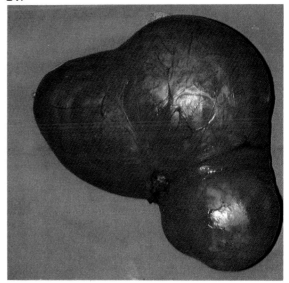

247   The broad ligament fibroid shown in **245** and **246** after its removal. It measured 24 cms × 17 cms × 11 cms and was partly cystic and partly solid. The solid portion comprised approximately 20% of the whole tumour. These features and the position of the tumour present difficulties when making an accurate pre-operative diagnosis. Microscopic examination revealed the tumour to be a benign leiomyoma showing widespread oedema and cystic degeneration.

248 A large serous cystadenoma exposed at operation. The other ovary can be seen to be normal in size.

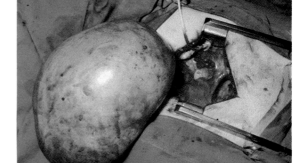

249 A serous cystadenocarcinoma. The appearances are not dissimilar to those shown in **248**. Unfortunately, histological examination revealed it to be malignant. There was no evidence of any spread elsewhere in the abdomen and the cyst wall had not been penetrated as far as could be ascertained.

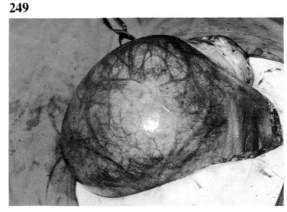

250 A benign dermoid cyst showing hair and skin-like tissue when opened.

251 A benign dermoid cyst showing a wide variation in its appearance on cross-section. Hair and fatty material are visible. These tumours are often bilateral. On examination these cysts feel solid and are often felt in front of the uterus. Whether or not this is due to their weight has not been established.

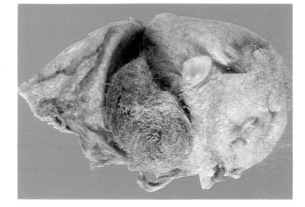

252 A solid ovarian tumour which proved to be a Brenner tumour. Incidental finding in a patient who attended for a cervical smear. Hence the importance of always carrying out a bimanual examination when taking a cervical smear.

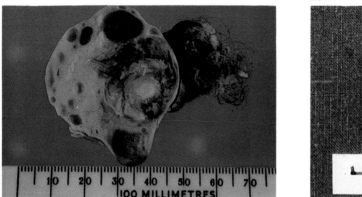

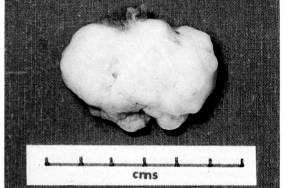

253

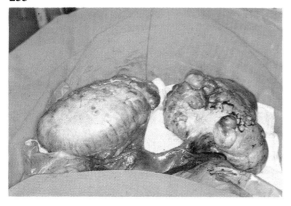

254

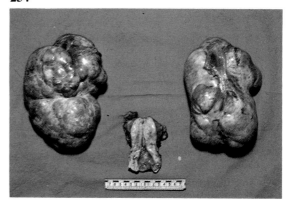

253 Bilateral papillary cystadenoma which proved to be benign. Fortunately, the patient had completed her family. A total hysterectomy and bilateral salpingo-oophorectomy was carried out.

254 Bilateral adenocarcinoma of the ovary in a post-menopausal woman. Her only complaint was of abdominal swelling and slight discomfort. Unfortunately, the patient died within 12 months of their removal. Note the size of the ovarian tumours compared with the uterus.

255

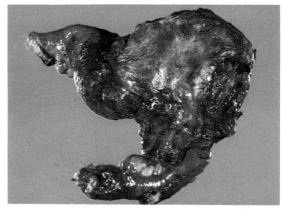

255 Endometriosis of the ileum. The patient, who had had endometriosis for years, presented with all the signs and symptoms of intestinal obstruction. Laparotomy revealed the site of the obstruction to be in the ileum. The specimen shows a 20 cm length of ileum, part of which is dilated and shows muscle hypertrophy. The other part forms a circular loop which is adherent to the distended part by dense fibrosis. Histologically there was endometriosis in the submucosa, muscularies and serosa.

256

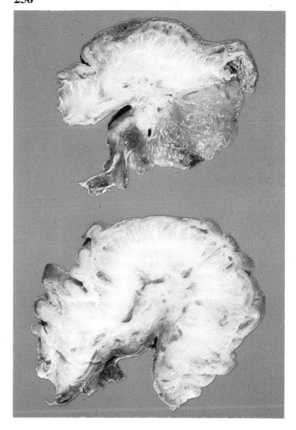

256 Endometriosis of the colon. In this case, the obstructive lesion had mimicked a carcinoma. Subsequent to resection this patient was maintained on hormone therapy to suppress ovulation without further problems for 15 years.

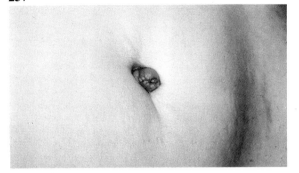

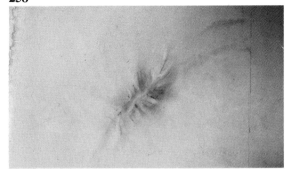

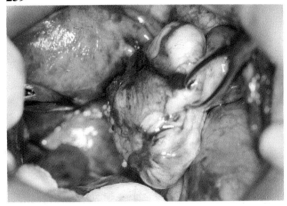

257 Endometriosis of the umbilicus. The picture being taken with the patient on her side.

258 Endometriosis in a scar. Implantation from an operation in which the uterine cavity is opened. The striae confirm that this patient had been parous. An operation likely to be followed by this condition, as was in this case, is a legal abortion by hysterotomy.

259 Endometriosis of the ovary. The ovary has been freed from its adhesion and multiple small endometriotic cysts are visible below the forceps. There is a larger one above the forceps. The forceps have ruptured one of the endometriotic cysts and the typical 'chocolate' material is visible.

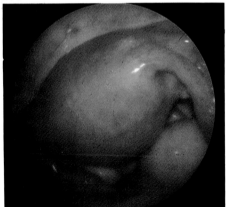

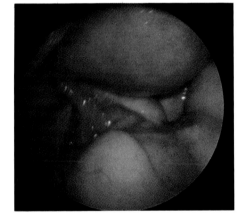

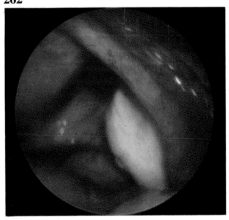

260 Laparoscopy view of the pelvic organs. The uterus is visible with the inner part of the right fallopian tube. The outer part of the left tube and the left ovary are visible in the lower part of the picture.

261 Laparoscopy. A closer view of the left fallopian tube and ovary. The fundus of the uterus is in the upper part of the picture, and bowel is present in the lower part of the picture.

262 Laparoscopy. The right ovary in view, partly covered by the fallopian tube. The uterus is in the upper left part of the picture.

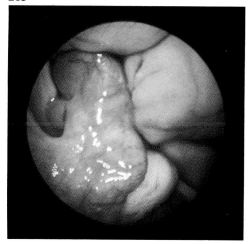

263 Laparoscopy hydrotubation. The methylene blue dye is visible in the fallopian tube which is slightly distended by the dye. Part of the ovary is visible on the left of the picture and the bowel is also seen in the lower part of the picture, and on the right.

264 Laparoscopy hydrotubation. Dye is present in the Pouch of Douglas plus spill anteriorly. The fundus of the uterus is in the middle of the picture.

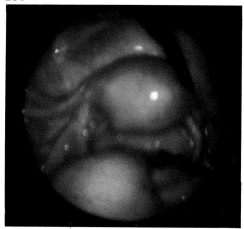

265 Mullerian duct failure. An unexpected finding at the time of hysterotomy operation. The patient had no problems in conceiving or in pregnancy, or labour. She had four children. There had been failure of one Mullerian duct to develop and a subsequent IVP revealed only one kidney on the same side as the Mullerian duct development.

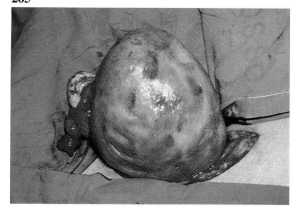

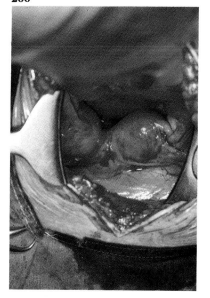

266 Failure of fusion of Mullerian duct. This patient had two vagina, two cervices and two uteri. Each uterus having a single tube.

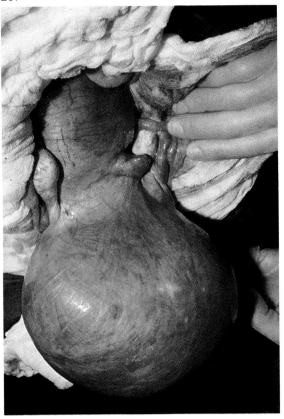

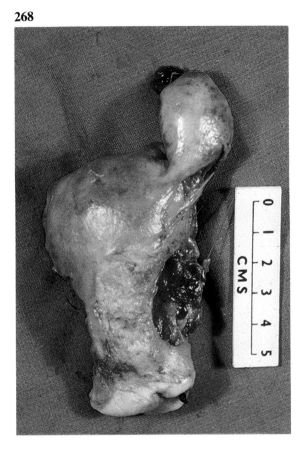

267 Leiomyosarcoma. Macroscopic appearances would suggest a large fibroid uterus with posterior wall fibroids. Unfortunately, microscopic examination revealed the accepted, but rare, complication of sarcomatous change.

268 Traumatic rupture of the uterus. The site of rupture is apparent in the right side of the uterus.

269

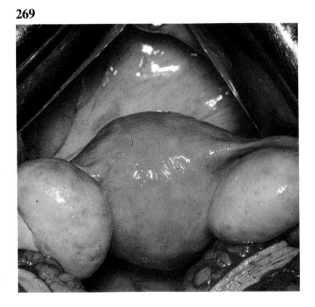

269 Polycystic ovaries Typical appearances of smooth, large white ovaries. This patient complained of infrequent periods and infertility.

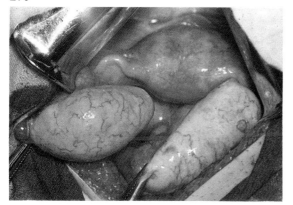

270 Polycystic ovaries. Less typical appearances. Vessels are seen on the enlarged smooth ovaries.

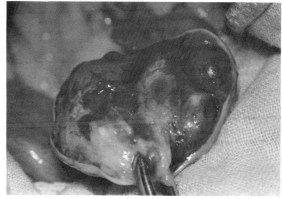

271 Polycystic ovary. One of the ovaries shown in **270** on incising the ovary. Multiple large cysts.

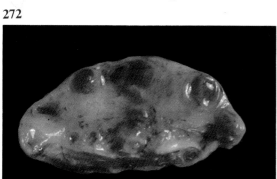

272 Polycystic ovary. The appearance of a cross-section of ovary. The cystic follicles were up to 6 mm in diameter and were, on microscopic examination, found to be in various stages of involution. There were primordial follicles present but no corpora albicans seen.

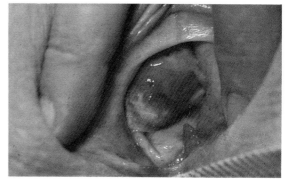

273 Secondary tumour from carcinoma of the endometrium. Two years after a total hysterectomy and bilateral salpingo-oophorectomy, the patient complained of vaginal discharge and bleeding. The presence of recurrent tumour in the lower part of the anterior vaginal wall is a recognised site. The commonest site is the vaginal vault. This patient did not have radiotherapy after her original operation.

274 Pelvic wall malignant lymph node. Exposure of the right pelvic wall at the time of a Wertheim's hysterectomy, using an extraperitoneal approach to expose the pelvic side wall. The external iliac artery and vein are visible on the right side. The ureter is held back by tape to help identification of its position in relation to the internal iliac vessels, which are close by. The enlarged nodes have been partially freed from their position in the bifurcation of the internal and external iliac vessels.

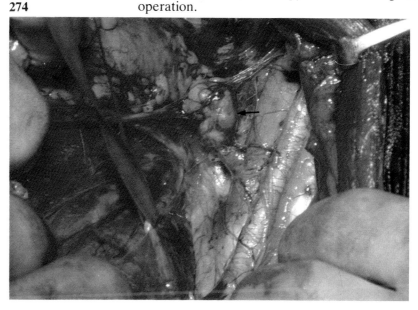

Early pregnancy and its complications

In the reproductive era one must always suspect pregnancy or a complication of pregnancy. The earliest clinical sign of pregnancy may be the vascularity of the breast. Diagnosis of an early pregnancy is often difficult, but in normal circumstances a further examination in four weeks will usually establish the diagnosis. In certain cases, as, for example, those who had had recurrent abortions, it may be helpful to have early confirmation of the diagnosis of pregnancy in order that appropriate therapy or rest may be prescribed.

If pregnancy is established, it is also essential to know that it is in the uterus and not in an ectopic site. The onus is, therefore, on establishing that the pregnancy is intrauterine rather than the reverse. The introduction of ever-improving ultrasonic machines and pictures has been a consider-able asset in this respect, since they can help confirm the diagnosis of pregnancy, and also whether it is an intrauterine one. They can also ascertain that a pregnancy is continuing satisfactorily, or if there is an abnormality such as hydatidiform mole. The demonstration of uterine fibroids and ovarian cysts are an additional benefit whether the patient is pregnant or not.

If a patient aborts, the products should always be examined to determine: whether the trophoblastic tissue is normal or abnormal; whether there is an embryo or fetus or not; and, if present, that it is normal or abnormal.

Some aspects of early pregnancy are considered in this section, but should not be regarded as being complete. It also allows the opportunity to show the early fetus.

275 **Incomplete abortion**, placental tissue. No fetus present.

275

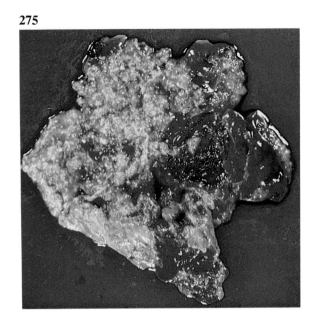

276

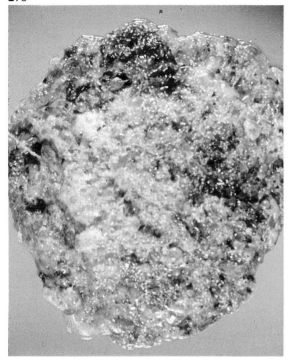

276 Hydatidiform mole tissue, typical picture, passed spontaneously when the patient aborted.

277

277 Hydatidiform mole tissue: a closer view. The cluster of vesicles are easily made out.

278

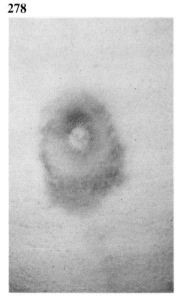

278 Cullen's sign. The bluish discolouration around the umbilicus in cases of intraperitoneal bleeding, especially ruptured ectopic gestation.

279

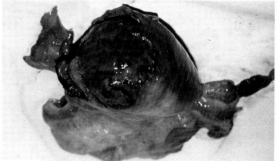

279 Ectopic gestation in the fallopian tube. A blood clot is visible at the site of rupture. There were over four pints of blood in the abdomen.

280

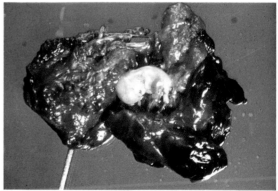

280 Ectopic gestation sac opened with fetus exposed from the surrounding trophoblastic tissue and blood clot.

281

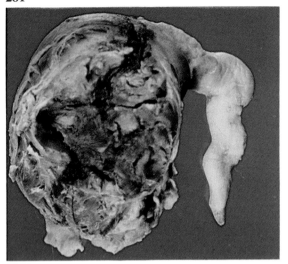

281 Tubal pregnancy with rupture and extrusion of fetus through the tube. The partly organised tissue and part of the fallopian tube are visible.

282

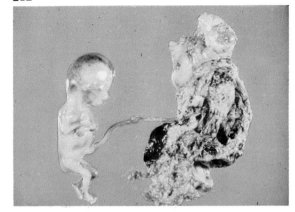

282 Spontaneous abortion with placental tissue and fetus.

283

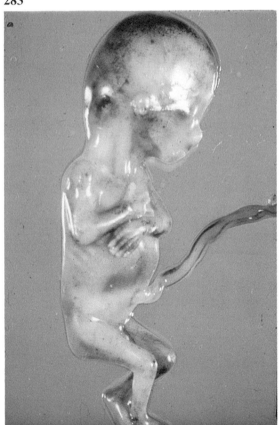

283 The fetus in the previous picture shown in more detail. Well-formed and developed.

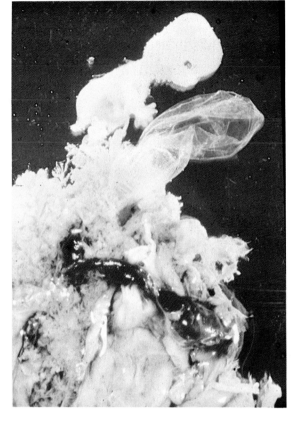

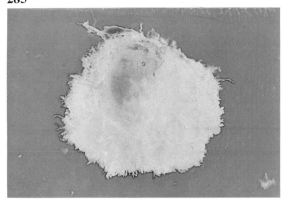

284 Products of conception from an abortion. The limb bud of the fetus and the ruptured sac are visible.

285 A complete sac with fetus visible inside the membranes. It is always important to examine the products passed. This allows the trophoblastic tissue to be inspected to exclude a hydatidiform mole. The presence of an embryo or fetus is important since it excludes a blighted ovum. If the fetus is big enough it may be possible to exclude major abnormalities especially of the central nervous system.

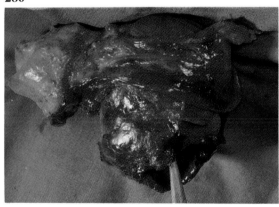

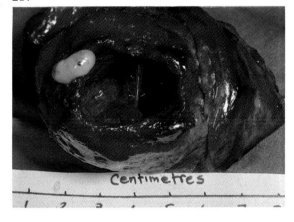

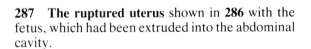

286 A ruptured uterus with a pointer showing the rupture site.

287 The ruptured uterus shown in **286** with the fetus, which had been extruded into the abdominal cavity.

288 The fetus adjacent to the ruptured portion of the uterus in lateral view.

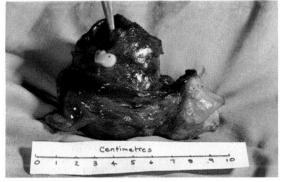

289 Septic abortion: postmortem findings in a patient with septic abortion; paralytic ileus and gangrene of the bowel.

289

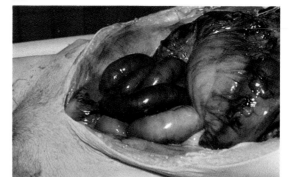

290

290 An ultrasonic scan of a 3 week gestation sac. The ultrasonic scan can pick up an early sac before pregnancy tests are positive, especially if the bladder is full at the time of examination. The sac is seen in the centre of the picture.

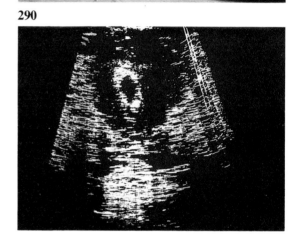

291

291 A blighted ovum shown on ultrasonic scan. No fetal parts are seen in the gestation sac and there is a 'C' shaped appearance, as shown. This is due to a break in the gestation sac.

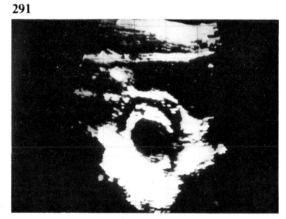

292

292 An early pregnancy with an IUCD in position. IUCD's are shown on scan as conspicuous echoes within a uterine cavity. The positions of the bladder (1), the cervix (2), and intra-uterine contraceptive device (3) are indicated.

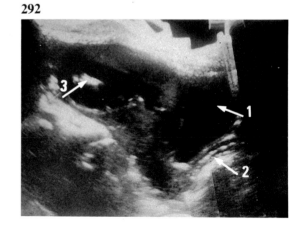

293 **A complete abortion** with the cervical canal open. The positions of the uterus (1), cervix (2) and vagina (3) are shown.

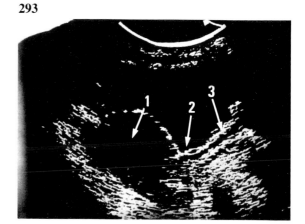

294 **Hydatidiform mole:** typical appearance on an ultrasonic scan of a series of echoes giving a classical 'snowstorm' appearance.

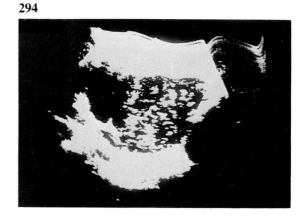

295 **A pregnancy with an ovarian cyst** shown by ultrasonic scan. The positions of the bladder (1), ovarian cyst (2) and gestation sac (3) are shown. The commonest cyst in early pregnancy is a corpus luteum of pregnancy.

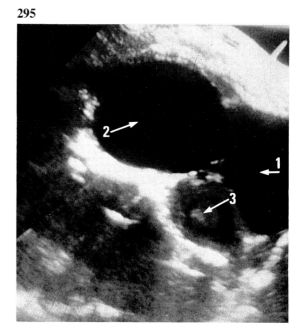

Miscellaneous conditions

The condition or syndromes dealt with in this section are those which did not fit easily into the other sections. Some conditions are rarely encountered in normal practice, and these cases are often referred to a few acknowledged experts. Some are problems of intersex, whilst others have major upsets of other systems and the gynaecological problem(s) are, by comparison, minor. The effect(s) on the genital tract may be reversed by appropriate systemic therapy. In other instances, the inability to conceive is the real reason for referral of the patient to the gynaecologist. The investigation and management of infertility is not appropriate for this type of book. It is dealt with in standard text books of gynaecology. Dermatological conditions and sexually transmitted diseases are associated with gynaecological problems and an example of each of these conditions is included in this section.

296

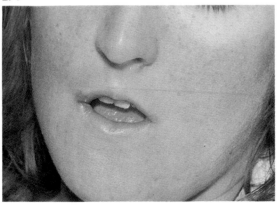

296 The Stevens-Johnson disease or syndrome. A condition in which there is erythema multiforme with a purulent conjunctivitis, which is often complicated by corneal ulceration and perforation. It is associated with fever and stomatitis (vesicles in the mouth, nose, genito-urinary orifices and anal canal). The face shows a slight rash with small vesicles below the left nostril on the mouth.

297

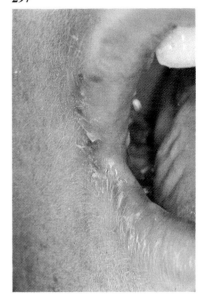

297 Stevens-Johnson disease. A closer view of changes at the angle of the mouth.

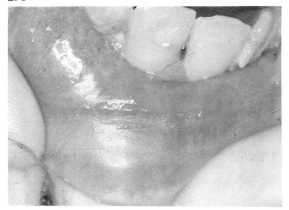

298 Stevens-Johnson disease. Effect on lip and gums. Vesicles between the teeth.

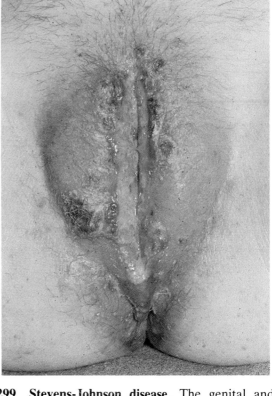

299 Stevens-Johnson disease. The genital and anal effects. The vesicles have, in most places, broken down with scar formation, but some are still visible.

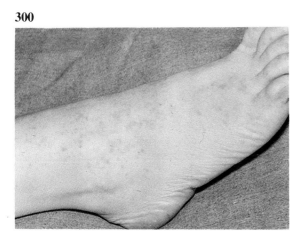

300 Stevens-Johnson disease. The erythema multiforme is easily visible on the dorsum of the foot and lower part of the leg.

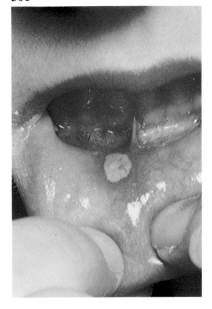

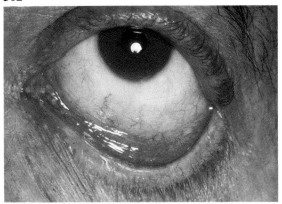

301 Behcet's syndrome: lip ulcer. Note erythematous margin.

302 Behcet's syndrome. Recurrent oral and genital ulceration, plus recurrent iridocyclitis from Behcet's syndrome. This patient developed an iridocyclitis after she had had episodes of oral and genital ulceration. The appearance of the eye represent iridocyclitis.

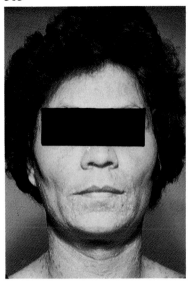

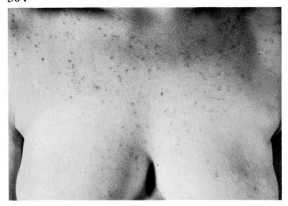

304 Secondary syphilitic rash. A view of the chest, which shows the rash to be symmetrical in distribution. The rash was evenly distributed over the back. It was non-irritant and did not trouble the patient.

303 Secondary syphilitic rash. Front view of the head and neck.

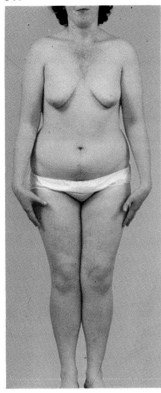

305 Familial hirsutism. This patient complained of excessive hair on her face, body and legs. She had no other complaints. Her menstrual cycle was normal and she had been pregnant. All investigations were negative except for the fact that female relatives were also hirsute.

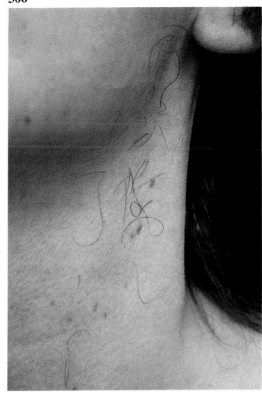

306 Familial hirsutism. A view of the side of the neck of the patient shown in **305**.

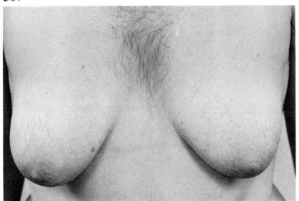

307 Familial hirsutism. Excessive hair growth between breasts. There are also long hairs on the breasts.

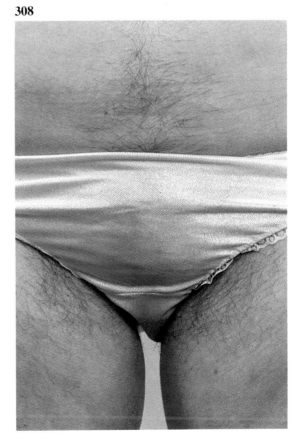

308 Familial hirsutism. Masculine type of hair distribution on abdomen and inner aspects of thighs.

309

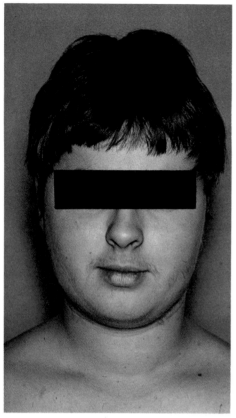

310

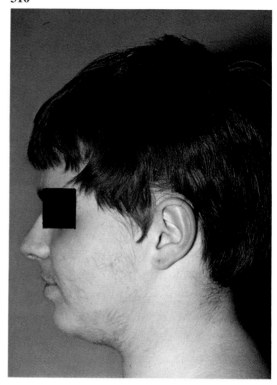

310 Hirsutism associated with Stein-Leventhal syndrome. Side view of the patient shown in **309**.

309 Hirsutism associated with Stein-Leventhal syndrome. Marked hirsutism of the face, especially the upper lip. This patient had infrequent periods and complained of infertility.

311

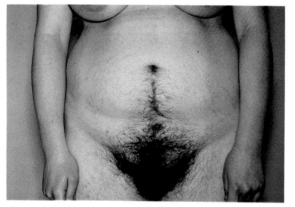

312

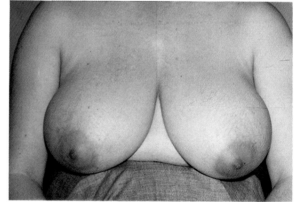

311 Hirsutism associated with Stein-Leventhal syndrome. The male type of distribution on the abdomen. Less marked on the forearms.

312 Hirsutism associated with Stein-Leventhal syndrome. The breasts of this patient with Stein-Leventhal in many respects suggest pregnancy changes. In fact, on two occasions when there had been prolonged periods of amenorrhoea, she had been presumed to be pregnant on the appearance of her breasts. This is not uncommon in these patients.

313

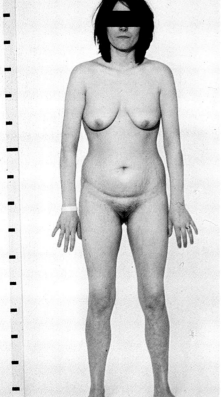

313 Hypopituitarism. This patient had developed Sheehan's syndrome following a severe postpartum haemorrhage. The ischaemic necrosis of the anterior pituitary had not been complete. She had lethargy and amenorrhoea. Investigations revealed that she was hypothyroid.

314

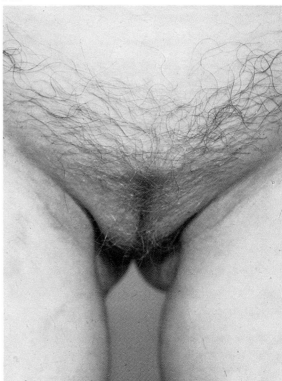

314 Hypopituitarism: Sheehan's syndrome. This patient had lost some weight but was not cachexic. There was loss of hair and some genital atrophy. The early changes in the pubic region for the patient in **313** are shown.

315 Galactorrhoea. A history of galactorrhoea is often found in patients with amenorrhoea and, or, infertility if sought. It is often due to an excess of prolactin secretion. It can also be caused by various drugs or excessive manipulation.

315

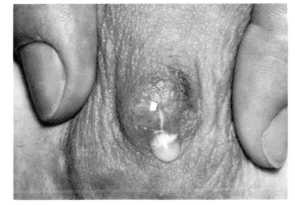

316

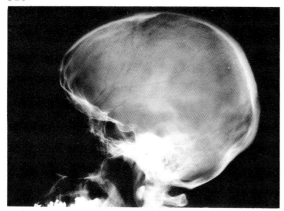

316 Lateral skull X-ray: in the investigation of amenorrhoea and infertility with hyperprolactinaemia, X-rays of the pituitary fossa are carried out. It can be normal, enlarged or have a normal variation.

318

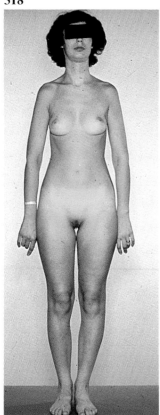

318 Testicular feminisation syndrome. A woman with well-developed breasts and minimal pubic hair. Chromosome arrangement 46 XY and chromatin negative buccal smear.

320 Testicular feminisation. The gonads (testes) removed from the patient shown in **318** and **319**. The testes were intra-abdominal.

317

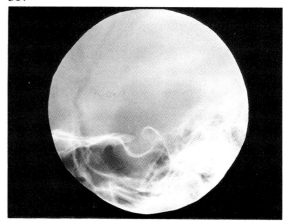

317 Pituitary fossa. A closer view of the pituitary fossa shown in **316** reveals a double floored pituitary fossa. There was no abnormality of pituitary function but sometimes tomograms are required to determine whether or not the pituitary fossa is normal.

319

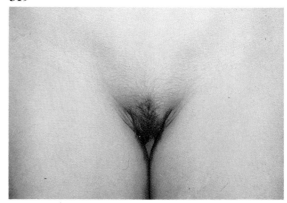

319 Testicular feminisation. A well-developed vulva, but scanty pubic hair. There are no signs of the scars from a hernia repair operation. A high proportion of these individuals develop hernias in childhood.

320

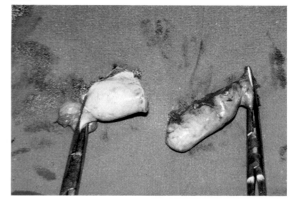

321 Turner's syndrome (45 chromosomes [XO]). The picture on the left shows the patient before oestrogen therapy. Her complaint was, as usual primary amenorrhoea and failure to grow as much as other girls of her age. The picture on the right was taken two years later when there had been no further increase in height and oestrogen therapy had been given for six months. There is cubitus valgus present in both forearms.

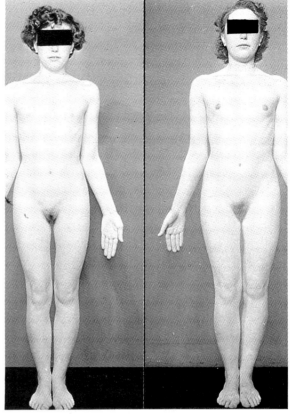

321

322 Atypical Turner's syndrome. This patient was 162.6 cm (5′ 4″) in height. One of the commonest forms of mosaicism in Turner's syndrome is sex chromatin positive gonadal dysgenesis (XO/XX mosaic). This was the reason for this patient's gonadal dysgenesis. The secondary sex characteristics were reasonably well developed despite her prime symptoms of amenorrhoea and infertility.

323 Gonadal dysgenesis. A side view of the patient shown in **322**.

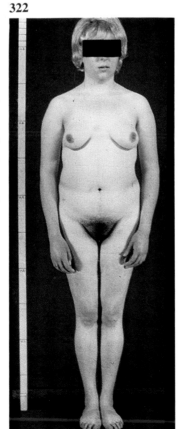

322

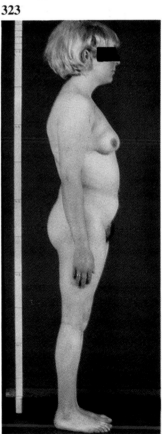

323

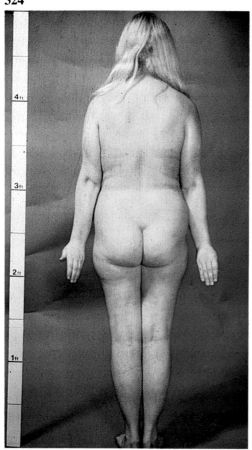 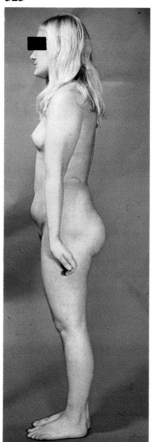

324 Gonadal dysgenesis. Another XO/XX mosaic. Height 149.9 cm (4′ 11″) and a cubitus valgus (increased carrying angle of the arms) on viewing from the back. This patient had streak ovaries.

325 Gonadal dysgenesis. A side view of the patient shown in **324**.

326 Turner's syndrome. Despite the Cushing-like appearance, this patient was a typical Turner's syndrome (45 chromosome XO). It is not surprising that she was initially referred as a possible Cushing's syndrome.

327 Turner's syndrome. The side view of the patient shown in **326**.

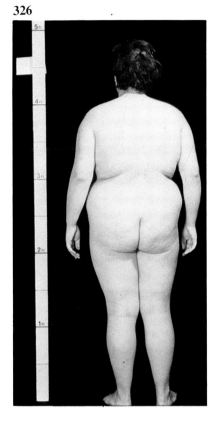
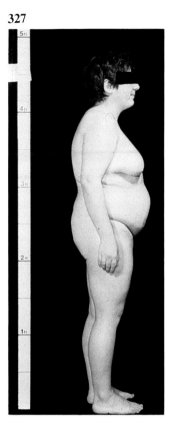

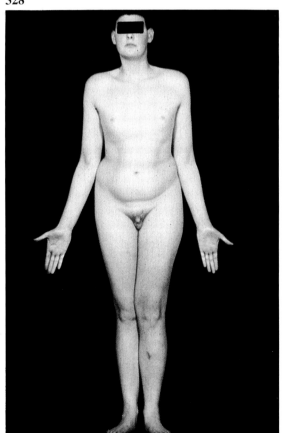

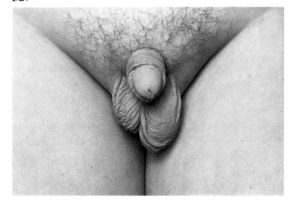

328 Klinefelter's syndrome (47 XXY). The typical picture of a tall, eunuchoid individual with poor development of the genitalia.

329 Klinefelter's syndrome. Showing the small genitalia. In this case, the testes have descended and are small; the right being extremely small, and the left, on palpation, less than a third of the normal size.

330

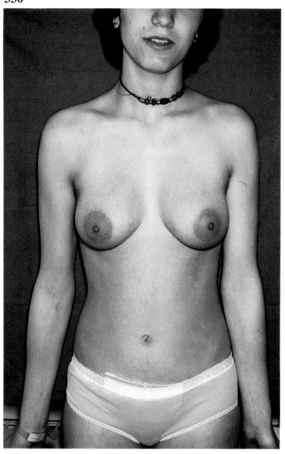

330 Uncertain sex: Female? This patient had been brought up as a female. There are obvious female secondary sex characteristics as can be observed by the breasts.

331 Uncertain sex: Male? A vagina and an enlarged clitoris. Chromosome pattern 46, XY.

332 Uncertain sex. The clitoris elevated to show the vagina.

331

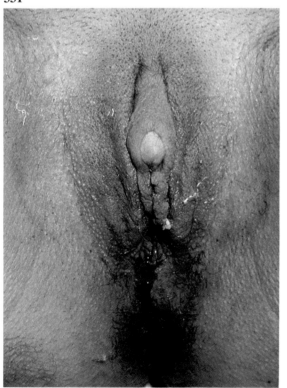

332

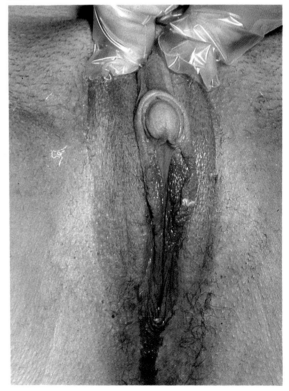

333 Streak gonad. One of the gonads of the patient shown in **330–332**.

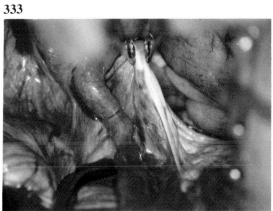

334 Mullerian duct and gonad. The other gonad from the patient shown in **330–333**. There is no formed uterus.

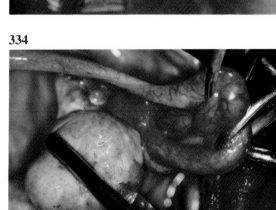

335 Gonad and Mullerian ducts. A more complete view of the enlarged gonad.

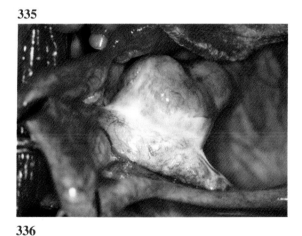

336 The gonads and Mullerian ducts. The specimen removed. Histologically the gonads were respectively a streak and a dysgerminoma.

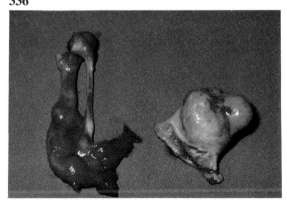

337

338

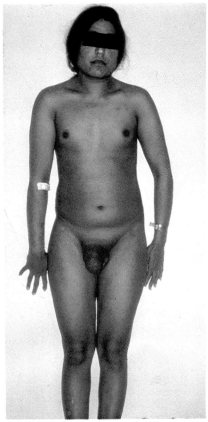 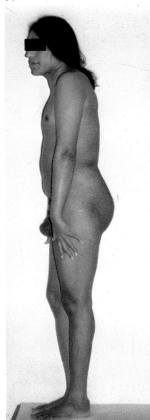

337 & 338 Male pseudohermaphrodite. This patient had been brought up as a female. The side view of the patient is less characteristic of a female, with poor breast development and suggestion of a male type phallus.

339

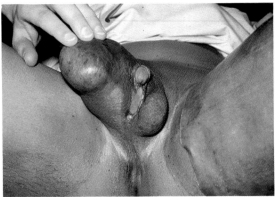

339 Male pseudohermaphrodite. The genitalia in more detail. Male type of genitalia with hydrocele on the right side.

340

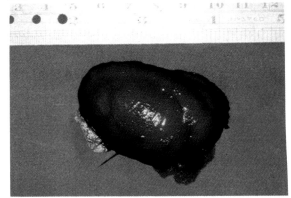

340 Male pseudohermaphrodite. The left gonad of the patient shown in **337–339**.

341

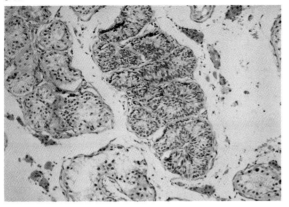

341 Male pseudohermaphrodite. Histological appearance of the gonad from the patient shown in **337–339**. A group of tubules with Sertoli's cell type of epithelium.

342

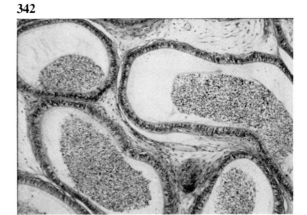

342 Male pseudohermaphrodite. Epididymis with spermatozoa from gonad removed from the patient shown in **337–339**.

343 & 344 Male pseudohermaphrodite. Front and side view. The appearance of the patient two months after reconstructive surgery and removal of testes. The patient had been given oestrogen.

343

344

345

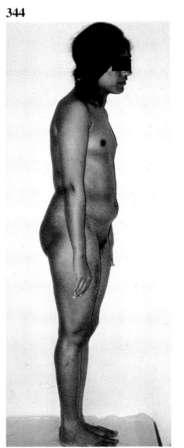

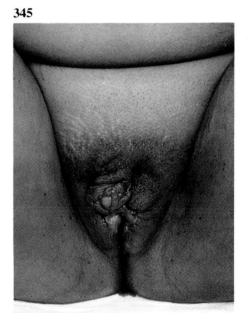

345 Male pseudohermaphrodite. The reconstructed genitalia two months after operation of the patient shown in **337–344**.

Colposcopy

The value of the colposcope apparatus is either overestimated' or underestimated. It provides additional information to the gynaecologist in a variety of conditions, and not only those related to the early diagnosis of cervical neoplasia. It is perhaps most useful in the continuing assessment of areas of abnormal epithelium, whether they are situated on the vulva, in the vagina, or in the cervix, over a period of time, often years.

The series of pictures that follow will, perhaps, give the reader an idea of the help that this apparatus can provide. The pictures that one obtains with different degrees of magnification are not the only source of information. The application of various solutions, plus the use of filters, allow abnormal vascular patterns to be demonstrated. Additional information is obtained from cytology and biopsies taken from the abnormal areas identified.

One might conclude by saying that there should be access to colposcopy facilities for every gynaecologist, but not every gynaecologist should have a colposcope. It is another area of gynaecological practice which should be in the hands of acknowledged experts. I am therefore particularly grateful to my colleague, Dr E Blanche Butler, MD, FRCOG, MRCPath, Senior Lecturer in Cytopathology, Department of Pathology, University of Manchester, for writing this particular section. The service that she and her team provide for all the consultants at St Mary's Hospital and for consultants in the North Western Region is, in my opinion, second to none.

Colposcopy
by Dr E. Blanche Butler

346   Normal cervix. *(× 16)* The squamocolumnar junction is seen and also the lower part of the endocervical canal because the bivalve speculum causes the external os to open as well as the vagina. Note the grape-like appearance of the columnar epithelium. The cervix has been swabbed with saline before the picture was taken. Where relevant, the material used will be inserted after the picture title.

346

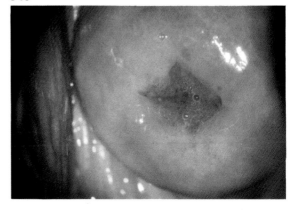

347   Ectopy showing early squamous metaplasia. *(Saline × 16)* Hormonal stimulation at puberty, during pregnancy and in some women on oral contraceptives causes eversion of the cervix so that more columnar epithelium presents in the vagina. This appearance was called a cervical erosion, but the term 'ectopy' is more correct as the columnar epithelium is intact and there is no ulceration. The acid pH of the vagina stimulates replacement of columnar epithelium by squamous epithelium and this process is called squamous metaplasia. It is at an early stage in this picture and the thin white metaplastic epithelium can be seen in the upper right quadrant of the ectopy.

347

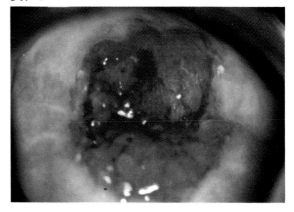

348 Normal transformation zone showing immature squamous metaplasia. *(2% acetic acid × 16)* When columnar epithelium is replaced by squamous epithelium the area is called the *'Transformation zone'*. This results in a new squamo-columnar junction being formed. The process is normal and occurs at some time in all women.

In this picture, the folds of columnar epithelium are disappearing under smooth, pink white squamous epithelium.

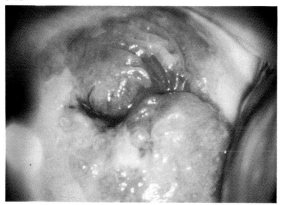

349 Normal healed transformation zone. *(Saline × 16)* The transformation zone is covered by mature metaplastic epithelium. Histologically this has the same appearances as original squamous epithelium, but it can be identified as metaplastic because of crypts lined by columnar epithelium which remain in the stroma. Note the new squamo-columnar junction. Crypt necks closed by squamous epithelium can usually be recognised as slightly raised rings on colposcopic examination.

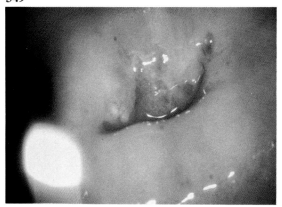

350 Pregnancy ectopy. *(2% acetic acid × 10)* In pregnancy there is often marked eversion of the cervix and hypertrophy of the endocervical folds. It can be difficult to demonstrate the squamo-columnar junction which is now well out on the cervix. Islands of immature squamous metaplasia are seen and stand out more clearly because the cervix has been painted with acetic acid.

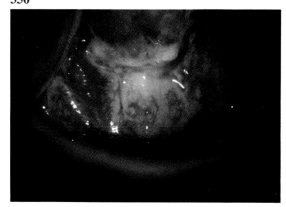

351 'Pill ectopy'. *(Saline × 10)* Some women on oral contraceptives show large ectopies similar to those seen in pregnancy. This is less common now that lower dose oestrogen preparations are used.

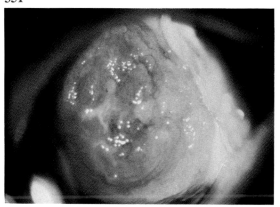

Illustrations **352–354** demonstrate the order of a colposcopic examination. In **352** the cervix has been cleaned with saline and a vascular transformation zone is seen. At higher magnification the vascular patterns can be recognised and these are shown in illustrations **355–358**.

352

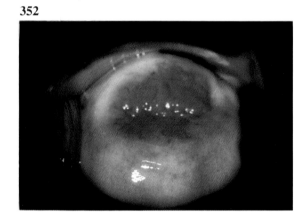

352 Atypical transformation zone. *(Saline × 10)* Most squamous carcinomas of the cervix develop in the transformation zone, probably due to the oncological effect of external factors such as virus infections or semen, on immature squamous epithelium. Cervical cytology screening permits the recognition of epithelial abnormalities before invasion occurs and cervical intra-epithelial neoplasia can be treated with excellent results. The colposcope is used to study the surface pathology of the cervix and to recognise the site and extent of abnormal epithelium.

353

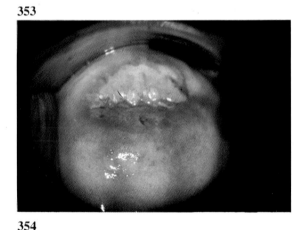

353 Atypical transformation zone. *(2% acetic acid × 10)* The cervix is painted with acetic acid and nuclear rich areas become white and opaque. Note the discrete dense white area on the anterior lip and compare this with the appearance of normal immature squamous metaplasia on the posterior lip.

354

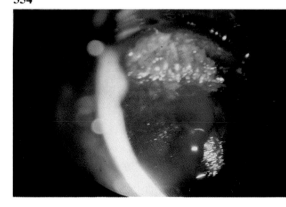

354 Atypical transformation zone. *(Schiller's iodine × 10)* The cervix is painted with Schiller's iodine. Mature squamous epithelium which contains glycogen stains a deep mahogany brown. Immature and abnormal epithelium which does not contain glycogen does NOT stain and such areas are called 'Schiller positive'. Note the yellow appearance of the discrete white area seen in **353**.

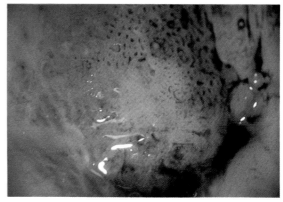

355 Atypical transformation zone: Punctation. *(Saline × 25)* Vascular patterns are studied after cleaning the cervix with saline. A green filter is used in the colposcope to show the vessels more distinctly. This picture shows punctation and in some areas the vessels reaching the surface are widely separated (coarse punctation). This patient was treated by cone biopsy and histology showed severe dysplasia (CIN III).

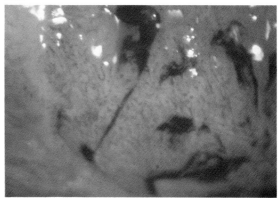

356 Atypical transformation zone: Punctation and mosaic. *(Saline × 25)* Some vessels are seen reaching the surface in the punctate pattern seen in **356**, but others surround islands of epithelium to give a mosaic pattern. There is greater irregularity of vessels in this picture which caused suspicion of an early invasive carcinoma, but histological sections showed carcinoma *in situ* (CIN III).

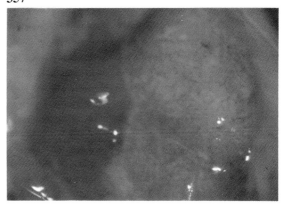

357 Atypical transformation zone: Irregular vessels. *(Saline × 40)* Complete irregularity of the vessels is seen with corkscrewing and variable calibre. The patient had an adenocarcinoma of the cervix (see **388**).

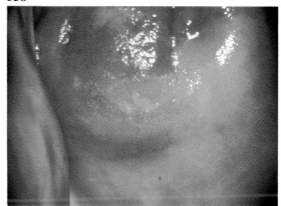

358 Atypical transformation zone: CIN III. *(Saline × 16)* Discrete areas of slightly thickened abnormal epithelium are seen and areas of punctation and mosaic can be recognised. Severe dysplasia bordering on carcinoma *in situ* was seen in histological sections (CIN III).

359 Atypical transformation zone: Microinvasion. *(Saline × 10)* A green filter has been used. A small punched out ulcer is seen to the right of the external os. Histological sections showed micro-invasion at the base of this ulcer.

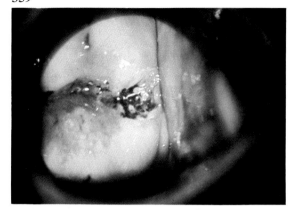

360 Atypical transformation zone: Squamous cell carcinoma. *(Saline × 16)* A green filter has been used. The external os is funnel shaped and a depressed area is seen just inside the posterior lip. The surface is roughened and there are irregularities of the vascular pattern. The presence of an invasive squamous cell carcinoma was confirmed on biopsy.

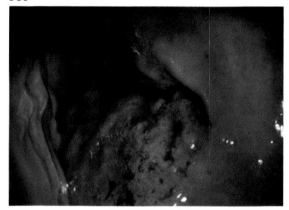

361 Squamous cell carcinoma. *(Saline × 16)* A slightly raised plaque of tumour surrounds the external os. It bleeds easily and the vascular pattern is irregular.

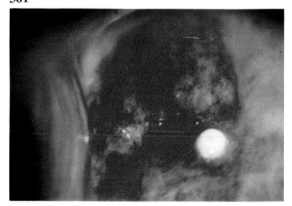

362 Procidentia with invasive carcinoma of the cervix. *(Saline × 10)* Unlike the previous examples this tumour was apparent on ordinary clinical examination. The picture shows the colposcopic view of the cervix using a green filter. The prolapse is not shown.

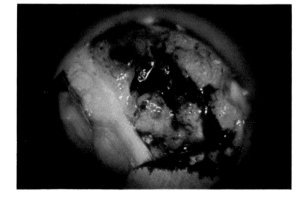

363 Squamous cell carcinoma of the cervix. *(Saline × 10)* This low-power view shows a depressed ulcer with an everted edge which replaces most of the anterior lip of the cervix.

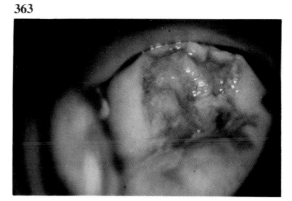

364 Squamous cell carcinoma of the cervix. *(Saline × 16)* At higher magnification vascular irregularity and areas of necrosis can be seen.

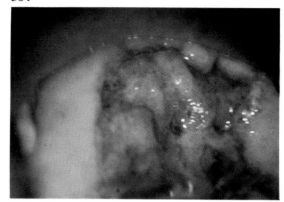

365 Residual carcinoma *in situ* at the vaginal vault. *(Saline × 10)* Following hysterectomy for carcinoma *in situ* (CIN III) this patient continued to have abnormal vault cytology smears. At this magnification, a vascular area can be seen at one cornu.

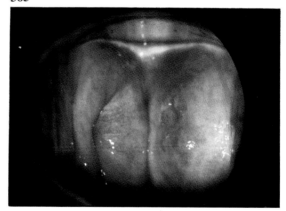

366 Residual carcinoma *in situ* at the vaginal vault. *(Saline × 40)* At a higher magnification the area is seen to have a discrete edge and a punctate vascular pattern. The area was excised and histological sections revealed carcinoma *in situ* (CIN III). Follow-up cytology was negative.

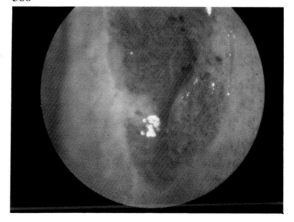

367 Granulation tissue at the vaginal vault following hysterectomy. *(Saline × 10)* This patient had an abdominal hysterectomy for adenocarcinoma of the endometrium. Following surgery she had two episodes of bleeding and a red area was noted at the vault at follow-up examination. This picture shows a vascular polypoidal structure with an irregular vascular pattern. The polyp was removed and histological sections showed that it consisted of granulation tissue. The vascular patterns seen in granulation tissue can be confused with the patterns seen with invasive tumour.

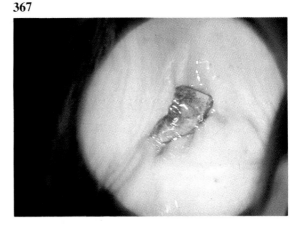

367

368 Slough following cryosurgery. *(Saline × 10)* This was the appearance of the cervix three weeks after cryosurgery.

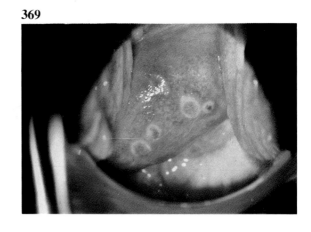

368

369 Decidual reaction on the cervix. *(Saline × 10)* Note the discrete white, disc like areas. Histological section of a biopsy from one of these areas showed thinning of the squamous epithelium over a focus of decidual reaction in the stroma.

369

370 Decidual reaction resembling an atypical transformation zone. *(2% acetic acid × 16)* Dyskaryotic cells were reported in the cervical smear. Colposcopy showed a large ectopy with a discrete aceto-white area at the periphery. Histological section of a biopsy showed a decidual reaction in the stroma and no evidence of dysplasia. Follow-up cytology was negative.

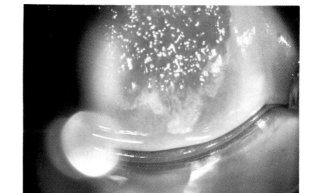

371 Herpes vesicles on the cervix. *(Saline × 16)* Note three small clear vesicles on the anterior lip of the cervix *(arrowed)*.

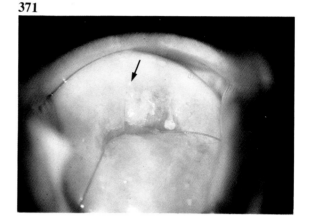

372 Condyloma on the cervix. *(Saline × 16)* A polyp like condyloma arises from the transformation zone on the posterior lip of the cervix. Note the dilated vessels indicating infection.

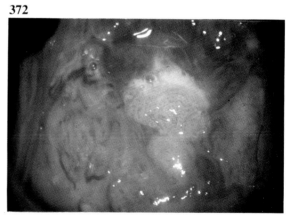

373 Condyloma on the cervix following renal transplant and immunosuppression. *(Saline × 16)* Green Filter. In this case the cervix was replaced by a large condyloma. Treatment was by excision. When last seen smaller condylomata were present on the vaginal wall. Immunosuppression can be associated with opportunist infections of which this is one example, due to papilloma virus.

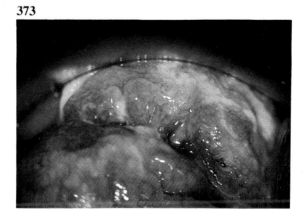

374 Multifocal warty lesions: Cervix. *(Saline × 10)* Hyperkeratotic warty lesions are seen on the portio of an otherwise normal cervix.

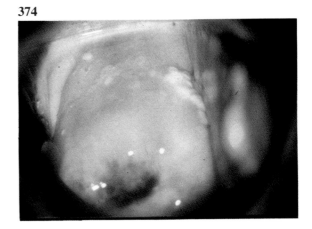

375 Multifocal warty lesions: Cervix. *(Schiller's iodine × 10)* This is the same case as **374** with the cervix painted with Schiller's iodine. The warty areas are demonstrated more clearly as the hyperkeratosis of the warty lesions prevents staining with Schiller's iodine.

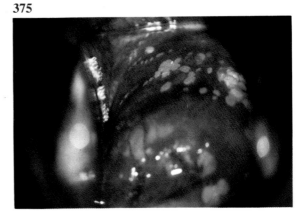

376 Multifocal warty lesions: Vulva. *(Saline × 16)* This is the same patient as **374** and **375**. Warts are also present on the perineum.

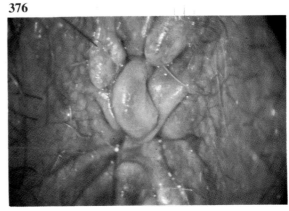

377 Multifocal condylomata: Cervix. *(Saline × 16)* Green Filter. A large condyloma is largely replacing the cervix. A green filter has been used to demonstrate the characteristic vascular pattern.

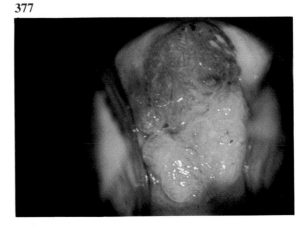

378 Multifocal condylomata: Urethra. *(Saline ×
16)* The same as **377**. A condyloma also arises at
the urethral orifice.

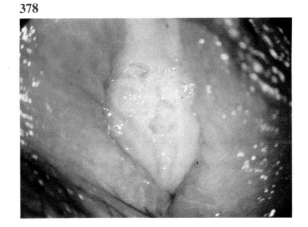

**379 Lichen sclerosis of the vulva in a child aged
9 years.** *(Saline. Portrait study)* White patches due
to hyperkeratosis are seen on the labia and on the
perineum.

Other vulval dystrophies have the same
appearance so biopsy is essential to establish the
nature of the lesion. This is illustrated by **46** in
which similar changes are seen in the vulva, but
histological sections show a multifocal microinvasive basal cell carcinoma.

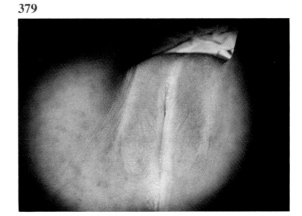

**380 Lichen sclerosis of the vulva in a child aged 9
years.** *(Saline × 16)* This is the same case as **379**
taken on another occasion. The thick white
epithelium on the inner surface of the left labium
majora is shown.

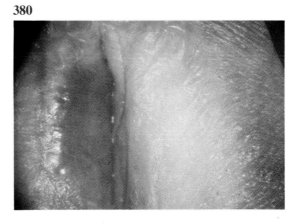

381 Recurrent squamous cell carcinoma of the vulva. *(Saline × 16)* A raised plaque of recurrent tumour is seen near the urethra. Note the irregular vascular pattern.

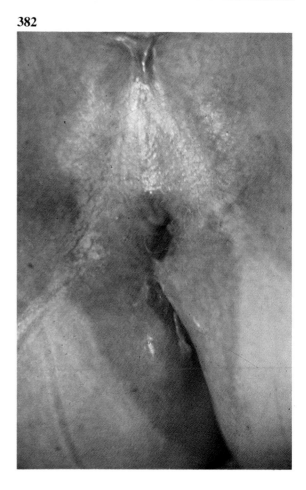

382 Recurrent carcinoma of the vulva. *(Saline. Portrait study)* The tissue is vascular and oedematous. Note the discrete deeper red area on the perineum.

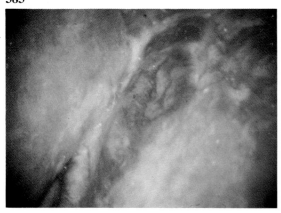

383 Recurrent carcinoma of the vulva. *(Saline × 16)* The same case as **382**. The discrete red area is shown through the colposcope and is now seen to be a depressed ulcer with areas of necrosis.

384 Malignant melanoma of the vulva. *(Saline × 6)* The labium minor at the introitus is distended by a tumour. Note the focal deposition of brown pigment.

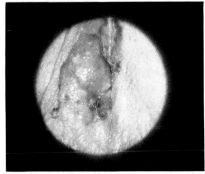

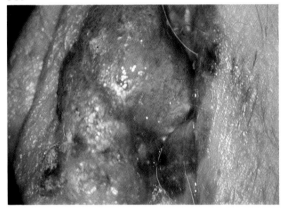

385 Malignant melanoma of the vulva. *(Saline × 16)* Green Filter. The same case as **384** seen at a higher magnification using a green filter. Pigment is seen more clearly. An abnormal vascular pattern is not seen in this case because of the thickness of the overlying epithelium.

385

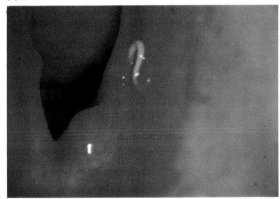

386 Vulvo-vaginitis due to Threadworm infestation. *(Saline × 25)* Note the threadworm which came out of the vagina in response to the heat of the colposcope lamp.

386

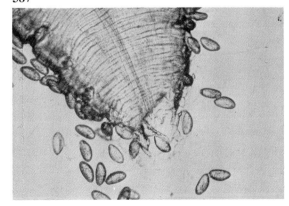

387 Threadworm. *(Photomicrograph)* The threadworm was caught and transferred to a microscope slide. The pressure of the cover slip has caused the ova to spill out of the body.

387

388 Adenocarcinoma of the cervix. *(Saline × 10)* This patient had an abnormality of the renal tract on the left side (double kidney, double ureters) and an adenocarcinoma on the left side of the cervix when aged 24. There had been no oestrogen exposure. The patient is alive and well six years after a Wertheim's hysterectomy. This tumour is shown at a higher magnification in **357**.

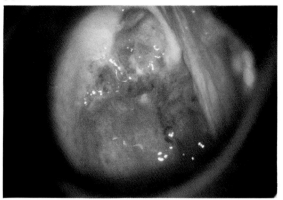

389 DES exposure in utero: Healed adenosis. *(Saline × 16)* The anterior fornix in a woman aged 22 years who had been exposed to diethylstilboestrol when in utero. Note the granularity of the epithelium. This probably reflects squamous metaplasia occurring in a columnar epithelium and it is unlikely that there will be any further sequelae.

389

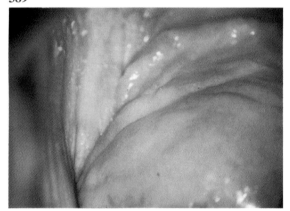

390 DES exposure: Adenocarcinoma of the vagina. *(Saline × 10)* This is a girl of 17 years-of-age who was exposed to diethylstilboestrol in utero. Tumour masses in the vaginal walls obscure the cervix. The tumour was multifocal in origin and the endocervical canal was not involved. **135** and **136** are photographs of this patient following five weeks progestogen therapy.

390

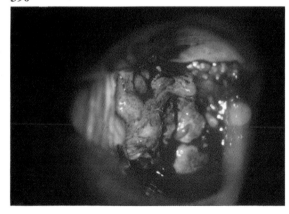

Index

Index

The references printed in **bold** type refer to picture and caption numbers, those in light type refer to page numbers.